AF182497

Neurofibromatosis - Diagnosis and Treatments

Edited by Lee Roy Morgan

Published in London, United Kingdom

Neurofibromatosis - Diagnosis and Treatments
http://dx.doi.org/10.5772/intechopen.1001529
Edited by Lee Roy Morgan

Contributors
Lee Roy Morgan, Branko Jursic, Marcus L. Ware, Tayler D. Payton, Marcus L. Ware, Shyam Patel, Thomas C. Chen, Frances E. Chow, Elisabetta Basso, Enrico Opocher, Franco Bassetto, Martina Grigatti, Alvise Montanari, Stefano Ferraresi, Federica Chiara, Vasiliy Korolishin, Yuri M. Poluektov

© The Editor(s) and the Author(s) 2023

The rights of the editor(s) and the author(s) have been asserted in accordance with the Copyright, Designs and Patents Act 1988. All rights to the book as a whole are reserved by INTECHOPEN LIMITED. The book as a whole (compilation) cannot be reproduced, distributed or used for commercial or non-commercial purposes without INTECHOPEN LIMITED's written permission. Enquiries concerning the use of the book should be directed to INTECHOPEN LIMITED rights and permissions department (permissions@intechopen.com).

Violations are liable to prosecution under the governing Copyright Law.

Individual chapters of this publication are distributed under the terms of the Creative Commons Attribution 3.0 Unported License which permits commercial use, distribution and reproduction of the individual chapters, provided the original author(s) and source publication are appropriately acknowledged. If so indicated, certain images may not be included under the Creative Commons license. In such cases users will need to obtain permission from the license holder to reproduce the material. More details and guidelines concerning content reuse and adaptation can be found at http://www.intechopen.com/copyright-policy.html.

Notice

Statements and opinions expressed in the chapters are these of the individual contributors and not necessarily those of the editors or publisher. No responsibility is accepted for the accuracy of information contained in the published chapters. The publisher assumes no responsibility for any damage or injury to persons or property arising out of the use of any materials, instructions, methods or ideas contained in the book.

First published in London, United Kingdom, 2023 by IntechOpen
IntechOpen is the global imprint of INTECHOPEN LIMITED, registered in England and Wales, registration number: 11086078, 5 Princes Gate Court, London, SW7 2QJ, United Kingdom

British Library Cataloguing-in-Publication Data
A catalogue record for this book is available from the British Library

Additional hard and PDF copies can be obtained from orders@intechopen.com

Neurofibromatosis - Diagnosis and Treatments
Edited by Lee Roy Morgan
p. cm.
Print ISBN 978-1-83769-580-5
Online ISBN 978-1-83769-579-9
eBook (PDF) ISBN 978-1-83769-581-2

We are IntechOpen, the world's leading publisher of Open Access books

Built by scientists, for scientists

6,400+
Open access books available

174,000+
International authors and editors

190M+
Downloads

156
Countries delivered to

Our authors are among the
Top 1%
most cited scientists

12.2%
Contributors from top 500 universities

CLARIVATE ANALYTICS BOOK CITATION INDEX INDEXED

WEB OF SCIENCE™

Selection of our books indexed in the Book Citation Index
in Web of Science™ Core Collection (BKCI)

Interested in publishing with us?
Contact book.department@intechopen.com

Numbers displayed above are based on latest data collected.
For more information visit www.intechopen.com

Meet the editor

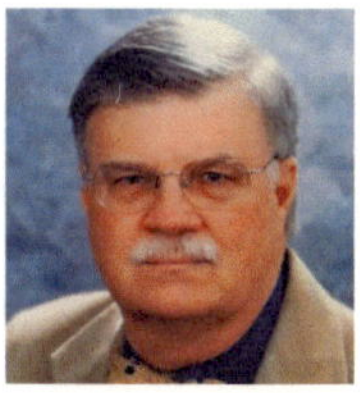

Lee Roy Morgan, MD, Ph.D., is a clinical pharmacologist and oncologist whose research interests are focused on the development of new and novel agents and devices that penetrate the CNS and spine and are effective therapies as treatment for both primary and metastatic malignancies involving the CNS. Dr. Morgan received his Ph.D. in Organic Chemistry from Tulane University, USA, in 1960. He completed post-doctoral studies at Imperial College, University of London, in 1961. In 1971, he received his MD from Louisiana State University Medical School, USA. From 1961 to 1986, he was professor and chairman, Department of Pharmacology, Louisiana State University Medical Center, USA. He is the founder, CEO, and medical director of DEKK-TEC, Inc., USA. Dr. Morgan is also an Adjunct Professor of Medicine, Tulane University School of Medicine and Adjunct Research Professor of Chemistry, University of New Orleans. From 1986 to 2015, Dr. Morgan was in oncology private practice in the New Orleans area. He has published more than 250 research articles, book chapters, and books. Dr. Morgan is married with four children and eight grandchildren.

Contents

Preface

Neurofibromatosis (NF) is a proliferative disorder that is inherited in an autosomal-dominant fashion and can involve cutaneous sites (skin), the nervous system, or gastric tissues. NF treatment is a medical challenge. Although there have been significant improvements in responses with the use of target-directed therapies in recent years, surgery and radiation remain the primary approaches to the management of NF. Advanced unresectable NF is commonly resistant to systemic therapies because of the lack of knowledge regarding the best mechanism(s) for drugs to penetrate the proliferative membranes.

The most common forms of NF are observed in the skin and nervous systems. NF type 1 (NF1) or von Recklinghausen's disease is an autosomal disorder caused by a loss of function mutation, either de novo or inherited, on the neurofibromin 1 (*NF1*) gene and presents with neurofibromatosis café-au-lait macules in the skin, freckles, and gliomas of the optic nerve. NF type 2 (NF2) has an autosomal dominant genetic pattern (loss of function mutation of the *NF* 2 gene) and presents as vestibular schwannomas and meningiomas.

NF1 accounts for about 96% of all NF cases with a prevalence of 1 in 3000 births. It occurs equally between gender and races. Fifty percent of patients have a spontaneous mutation, and the other half have an inherited mutation. There is 100% penetrance with variable expressivity. NF2 accounts for about 3% of all cases and has a prevalence between 1 in 33,000 births and 1 in 87,410 births.

Overall, long-term responses for NF have improved. However, there remains a paucity of useful therapeutic tools for the management of pediatric and adolescent patients with NF involving the CNS who are otherwise healthy but are seldom referred for clinical trials with novel new agents because they are younger than 18 years of age. Without new therapies, the management and support of pediatric and adolescent patients with CNS NF will remain inadequate; thus, more clinical research efforts in this area are badly needed. Only through new research endeavors and concepts are there possibilities of eradicating NF, especially NF involving the central nervous system.

Neurofibromatosis – Diagnosis and Treatment reviews recent developments in new approaches to NF diagnosis and treatment through neurocutaneous studies and collaborations, in-depth discussions, and reviews of diagnostic and therapeutic concepts that will improve the management and care of patients with NF-associated neurological challenges and disabilities.

'Each of us has been given the wisdom to reach our goals – just think about where we have been and where we are now – please do not stop!

It is an honor and pleasure to serve as editor for this volume. I hope that it will assist in bringing together clinicians, scientists, and researchers to investigate and develop new methods to improve the management of NF.

Lee Roy Morgan, MD, Ph.D.
CEO,
DEKK-TEC, Inc.,
New Orleans, LA, USA

Section 1

Introduction to Neurofibromatosis (NF)

Chapter 1

Introductory Chapter: Current Status of Neurofibromatosis – Diagnosis and Treatment

Lee Roy Morgan, Branko Jursic and Marcus L. Ware

1. Introduction

Neurofibromatosis (NF) is a group of genetic diseases that are associated with tumors that develop in the cutaneous and nervous systems. There are three types of neurofibromatosis that are each associated with unique signs and symptoms [1–3].

Neurofibromatosis type 1 (NF1) also known as von Recklinghausen disease causes skin changes (cafe-au-lait spots, freckling in armpit and groin area); bone abnormalities; optic gliomas; and tumors in the nerve tissue or under the skin. Signs and symptoms are usually present at birth. NF1 is the most common neurofibromatosis [1].

Neurofibromatosis type 2 (NF2) causes acoustic neuromas; hearing loss; ringing in the ears; poor balance; brain and/or spinal tumors; and cataracts at a young age [4].

Schwannomatosis (NF3) presents with schwannomas, pain, numbness, and weakness; it is the rarest type of NF [3].

All three types of NF are inherited in an autosomal dominant manner [1].

Every chapter in "Neurofibromatosis—Diagnosis and Treatment", reviews approaches to the diagnosis and treatment of NF through neurocutaneous studies, in-depth discussions, and/or reviews of diagnostic and therapeutic concepts that will improve the management and care of patients with NF-associated neurological challenges and disabilities.

2. Types of NF

NF is a rare genetic disorder. NF1 was originally characterized as the triad of polyostotic fibrous dysplasia of bone, precocious puberty, café-au-lait skin pigmentation, and associated endocrinopathies including hyperthyroidism, growth hormone excess, FGF23-mediated phosphate wasting, and hypercortisolism [1]. NF2 classically involves the nervous system—acoustic neuromas with hearing loss and optic gliomas—the McCune-Albright Syndrome (MAS) [1]. NF2 also induces bilateral acoustic neurofibromatosis and vestibular schwannoma neurofibromatosis [1, 3]. It is much less common than NF1 and is characterized by multiple tumors on the cranial and spinal nerves. Tumors that affect both of the auditory nerves and hearing loss beginning in the teens or early 20s are generally the first symptoms of NF2. Schwannomatosis (NF3) presents with schwannomas, pain, numbness, and weakness; it is the rarest type of NF [5].

The three types of neurofibromatosis (NF) are all proliferative disorders that are inherited in an autosomal dominant fashion, can involve cutaneous sites (skin), the nervous system or gastric tissues, and remain a medical challenge [1]. Although there have been significant improvements in responses with the use of target-directed therapies in recent years, surgery and radiation remain the primary approaches to the management of NF. Advanced unresectable NF is commonly 'resistant to systemic therapies' because of the lack of knowledge regarding best mechanism(s) for drugs to penetrate the proliferative membranes [6–9].

3. History

Records and reports of neurofibromatosis, as we currently appreciate the condition, were reported centuries ago [1]. The tumors and condition were first known as von Recklinghausen disease, the first person to describe NF [1]. There has been a slow improvement in the therapeutic approaches to the types of NF. The latter might only be associated with the improved quality of life available through support care only.

4. Histology

NF1 is usually associated with mutations on chromosome 17 with encoding of a cytoplasmic protein—neurofibromin. Neurofibromin is a tumor suppressor protein and regulator of cell proliferation signaling and differentiation. Neurofibromatosis (NF1) is a result of dysfunction or lack of neurofibromin, resulting in uncontrolled cell proliferation and tumor development (**Figure 1**) [1].

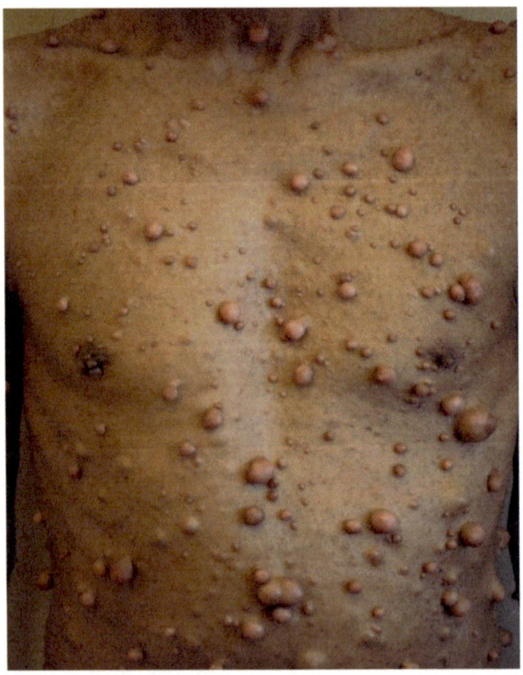

Figure 1.
Example of NF1.

The most common forms of NF are observed in the skin and nervous systems. NF1 or von Recklinghausen's disease is an autosomal disorder (caused by a loss of function mutation, either *de novo* or inherited, on the neurofibromin 1 gene and presents with café-au-lait macules in the skin, freckles, and gliomas of the optic nerve. Neurofibromin also binds to microtubules and has a role in the release of adenylyl cyclase, a cyclase involved in cognition, resulting in cognitive impairment [1].

NF1 tumors are usually benign arising from supporting Schwann nerve cell tissues but cause neurological damage by compressing nerves and other tissues [1].

NF type 2 (NF2) has an autosomal dominant genetic pattern (a loss of function mutation on chromosome 22). The mutation involves the Schwann cell genetic encoding of a cytoplasmic protein—Merlin [8]. Merlin regulates multiple growth factors, and its absence or during NF2 gene mutations, there are formation of tumors—vestibular schwannomas and meningiomas.

The latter results in bilateral acoustic neuromas involving the vestibulocochlear nerve or cranial nerve 8 and loss of hearing [8].

Schwannomatosis (NF3) has only recently been classified as a neurofibromatosis and involves mutations on Schwann cell SMARCB1 genes, resulting in spinal and peripheral nerve tumors in the perineal area [1]. The SMARCB1 gene and the chromosome 22 are different gene sites; however, mutations in both genes result in NF3 tumors. The SMARCB1 gene is located near the NF2 tumor suppressor gene, and thus, the original thoughts were that they were the same disease; the latter concept has been reversed [9].

5. Epidemiology

NF1 involves about 96% of all neurofibromatosis cases. Prevalence is 1 in 3000 births. It occurs equally between gender and races. Fifty percent (50%) of patients have a spontaneous mutation, and the other half have an inherited mutation. NF2 makes up about 3% of all cases and has a prevalence between 1 in 33,000 births with the disorder. The damage to nearby vital structures such as cranial nerves and brain tissue can be life treating [1].

NF3 is the rarest of the group (<1% incidence), and typically life expectancy is not affected in the latter patients with Schwannomatosis [1].

NF1 is the most common of the NF types and may be 'increasing in occurrence', but knowledge and management skills with the disease have improved, and presentations of the disease are not as prevalent; however, debilitation still exists—as noted above. Overall, long-term responses for NF have improved [1].

However, there remains a paucity of useful therapeutic tools and best approaches to therapy for pediatric and adolescent patients with NF involving the CNS, whom are otherwise healthy, but are seldom referred for clinical trials with novel new agents because they are <18 years of age.

6. Therapy: current and new

The neurofibromas that develop are usually initially benign, and surgical removal is optional—cosmetic, symptomatic, etc. However, for any neurological changes, new developments in sizes or progression to a malignant stage, a referral to a neurologist and/or surgeon is important [10, 11].

Treatment may include surgery, focused radiation, or chemotherapy. Acoustical and optic tumors may cause communication impairment and are often electively surgically removed. Monitoring for new signs of progressive neurological deterioration is mandatory, especially in the pediatric and adolescent aged group. Cataracts must be a considered a risk for all ages. Assessment for hearing impairment must be monitored for all ages [1–3].

Plexiform neurofibromas have malignant potentials (8–13% risk) and must be monitored closely—malignant tumors can develop peripherally in nerve sheaths [7].

Radiation can be used, but there is increased risk of malignant transformation [1].

Surgery to remove NF2 tumors completely is one option. Surgery for vestibular schwannomas does not restore hearing and usually reduces hearing. Sometimes surgery is not performed until functional hearing is lost completely. Surgery may result in damage to the facial nerve resulting in some degree of facial paralysis. Focused radiation of vestibular schwannoma is associated with a lower risk of facial paralysis than open surgery, but is more effective in shrinking small to moderate tumors than larger tumors [4, 8–10].

Chemotherapy with a drug that targets the blood vessels of vestibular schwannoma can reduce the size of the tumor and improve hearing, but some tumors do not respond at all, and responses are only temporary. Bone malformations can be corrected surgically, and surgery can also correct cataracts and retinal abnormalities. Pain usually subsides when tumors are removed completely [6, 9, 11].

In April 2020, the U.S. Food and Drug Administration approved selumetinib (Koselugo) as a treatment for children ages 2 years and older with NF1. The drug helps to stop tumor cells from growing [11].

Selumetinib (**Figure 2**) is a kinase inhibitor that is a selective inhibitor of the enzyme mitogen-activated protein kinase (MAPK kinase or MEK) subtypes 1 and 2. These enzymes are part of the MAPK/ERK pathway, which regulates cell proliferation (*i.e.*, growth and division) [11].

Imatinib mesylate has also been approved as treatment for plexiform neurofibromas in patients with neurofibromatosis type 1: a phase 2 trial [7, 11].

All drugs being used possess bio-releasable reactive halogenated moieties that could interact with DNA and interfere with genetic replication [7, 11].

In summary, the core therapeutic challenges to obtaining long-term objective responses include

- Transport of drugs into the tumor sheaths
- Although the use of protocols that include tumor target markers is becoming popular, the penetration of neurofibromas is still an issue.

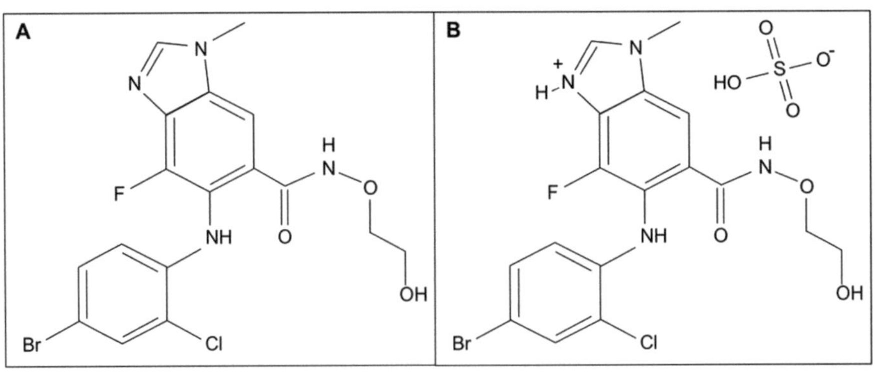

Figure 2.
A. Selumetinib (Koselugo) & B. Sulfate salt.

- For focal lesions, surgical resection followed by chemotherapy plus radiation
- The absence of Merlin protein is an issue. Studies with Merlin are of major interest for future clinical trials.
- Developing new drugs that are small or have unique transport mechanism(s)
- Identifying surface receptors on the affected nerve sheaths will assist with drug transport into the NFs.

7. Conclusion

This has been an attempt to review the history, pathology, and treatments available for neurofibromatosis. Minimal information is available regarding chemotherapy for the types of NF that are known; however, clinical trials are in progress worldwide. The positive responses observed and reported to date are support for continued clinical trials in neurofibromatosis.

Interesting chapters are presented in this book that review some of the progress being made that will allow improved management for this disease.

Abbreviations

NF1, NF2, NF3	Neurofibromatosis
SRS	Stereo-radiosurgery

Author details

Lee Roy Morgan[1]*, Branko Jursic[2] and Marcus L. Ware[3]

1 DEKK-TEC, Inc., New Orleans, Louisiana, USA

2 Department of Chemistry, University of New Orleans, New Orleans, Louisiana, USA

3 Department of Oncology Neurosurgery, Ochsner Medical Center, New Orleans, Louisiana, USA

*Address all correspondence to: lrm1579@aol.com

IntechOpen

© 2023 The Author(s). Licensee IntechOpen. This chapter is distributed under the terms of the Creative Commons Attribution License (http://creativecommons.org/licenses/by/3.0), which permits unrestricted use, distribution, and reproduction in any medium, provided the original work is properly cited.

References

[1] Kresak JL, Walsh M. Neurofibromatosis: A review of NF1, NF2, and Schwannomatosis. Journal Pediatrics and Genetics. 2016;**8**:234

[2] Ruggieri M, Iannetti P, Polizz A, et al. Earliest clinical manifestations and natural history of neurofibromatosis type 2 (NF2) in childhood: A study of 24 patients. Neuropediatrics. 2005;**36**:21-34

[3] MacCollin M, Chiocca EA, Evans DG, et al. Diagnostic criteria for schwannomatosis. Neurology. 2005;**64**:1838-1845

[4] Evans DG. Neurofibromatosis type 2 (NF2): A clinical and molecular review. Orphanet Journal of Rare Diseases. 2009;**4**:16

[5] Mathieu D, Kondziolka D, Flickinger JC, et al. Stereotactic radiosurgery for vestibular schwannomas in patients with neurofibromatosis type 2: An analysis of tumor control, complications, and hearing preservation rates. Neurosurgery. 2007;**60**:460-470

[6] Neurofibromatosis. Conference statement. National Institutes of Health Consensus Development Conference. Achieves of Neurology. 1988;**45**:575-578

[7] Robertson KA, Nalepa G, Yang FC, Bowers DC, Ho CY, Hutchins GD, et al. Imatinib mesylate for plexiform neurofibromas in patients with neurofibromatosis type 1: A phase 2 trial. The Lancet Oncology. 2012;**3**:1218-1224

[8] Plotkin SR, Merker VL, Halpin C, et al. Bevacizumab for progressive vestibular schwannoma in neurofibromatosis type 2: A retrospective review of 31 patients. Otology & Neurotology. 2012;**33**:1046-1052

[9] Ferner RE, Huson SM, Thomas N, Moss C, Willshaw H, Evans DG, et al. Guidelines for the diagnosis and management of individuals with neurofibromatosis 1. Journal of Medical Genetics. 2007;**44**:81-88

[10] Hirbe AC, Gutmann DH. Neurofibromatosis type 1: A multidisciplinary approach to care. Lancet Neurology. 2014;**13**:834-843

[11] Anderson MK, Johnson M, Thornburg L, Halford Z. A review of Selumetinib in the treatment of Neurofibromatosis type 1—Related plexiform Neurofibromas. The Annals of Pharmacotherapy. 2022;**56**:716

Section 2

Literature Review

Chapter 2

Neurofibromatosis Type 2: Case Presentation and Review of the Literature

Tayler D. Payton and Marcus L. Ware

Abstract

Patients diagnosed with neurofibromatosis type 2 (NF2) are likely to develop vestibular schwannomas, meningiomas, and other tumors that may be difficult to treat. These tumors and their locations can pose unique challenges for patients, caregivers, and medical providers. We describe a case of a patient with NF2 who presented with multiple tumors including bilateral vestibular schwannomas and multiple meningiomas. This case highlights the medical and surgical complexity of care of patients with NF2 and the need for ongoing surveillance by a multidisciplinary medical team. We also provide a brief review of literature focusing on NF2 and its treatment.

Keywords: neurofibromatosis type 2, case studies, NF2, vestibular schwannomas, meningiomas

1. Introduction

Our patient is a 63-year-old gentleman with several weeks' history of drooling, dysarthria, and altered mental status. His relevant past medical history included a brain tumor that had been removed 10 years earlier at a local hospital (no records available). According to his family, the patient had a single follow-up visit after surgery and had done well since. On examination, the patient was confused; he was oriented to people, but not place or time. Cranial nerve examination was unremarkable except for dysarthria and slight tongue deviation to the left. He had severe ataxia with a positive Romberg sign. His neurological exam was otherwise normal. He had an MRI that showed small bilateral vestibular schwannomas and multiple meningiomas including a large tumor attached to the falx on the right, a large tumor in the occipital region, and a cerebellar tumor causing compression of the fourth ventricle (**Figure 1**). Given these findings, the patient was diagnosed with neurofibromatosis Type 2 (**Table 1**).

The patient's symptoms were clinically related to cerebral compression and hydrocephalus caused by his right occipital and large cerebellar tumor. He was offered surgical intervention. The patient underwent a combined right occipital and posterior fossa craniotomy for tumor removal. Pathological evaluation of both tumors showed WHO Grade I meningioma. His postoperative images showed excellent resection with

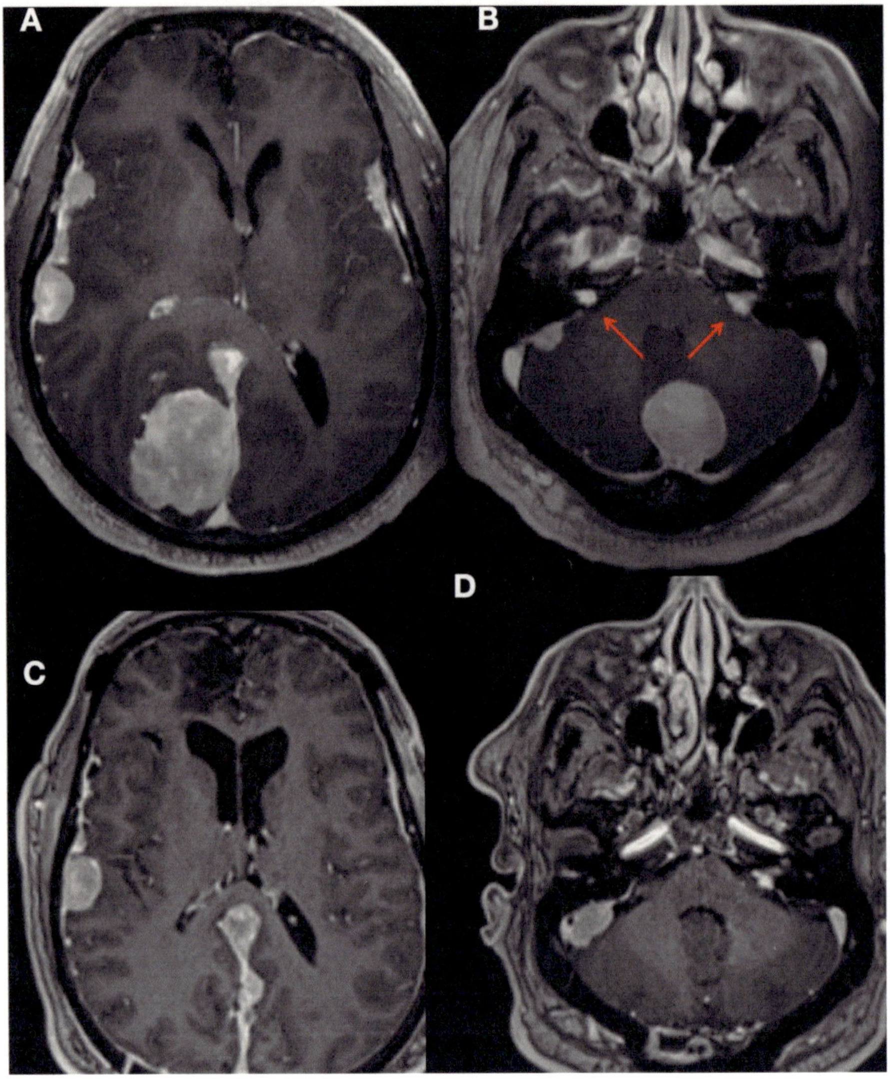

Figure 1.
Post-contrast T1-weighted MRI images in the axial orientation. Panel A shows a large meningioma that is attached to the posterior falx. Panel B shows a large meningioma attached to the dura of the posterior fossa. The arrows in this panel point to his vestibular schwannomas. Panels A and B show brain compression and narrowing of the right lateral ventricle in Panel A and 4th ventricle in Panel B. Panel C shows that the compression has been alleviated in the occipital area, and Panel D shows decompression in the posterior fossa. Panels A and B were performed before surgery. Panels C and D were performed 3 months after surgery.

good decompression (**Figure 1**). The patient did well postoperatively, and he returned to his normal level of function over the next 3 months. The patient was followed in our multidisciplinary CNS clinic every 4 months thereafter with an MRI of the brain with and without contrast.

One year after surgery, the patient began having difficulty with his balance and developed bilateral hand weakness. He had an MRI that showed compression of the foramen magnum with development of a cervical syrinx (**Figure 2**). The patient was offered and underwent a suboccipital craniectomy with C1 and C2 laminectomies and duroplasty to decompress his cerebellum and brainstem. The patient did well after surgery

1.	Bilateral vestibular schwannomas <70 years of age
2.	Unilateral vestibular schwannoma <70 years and a first-degree relative with NF2
3.	Any two of the following: meningioma, schwannoma (non-vestibular), ependymoma, cerebral calcification, cataract, and first-degree relative to NF2 or unilateral vestibular schwannoma and negative LZTR1 testing.
4.	Multiple meningiomas and unilateral vestibular schwannoma or any two of the following: schwannoma (non-vestibular), neurofibroma, glioma, cerebral calcification, and cataract
5.	Constitutional or mosaic pathogenic NF2 gene mutation from the blood or by the identification of an identical mutation from two separate tumors in the same individual.

Table 1.
Clinical criteria for NF2 [1, 2].

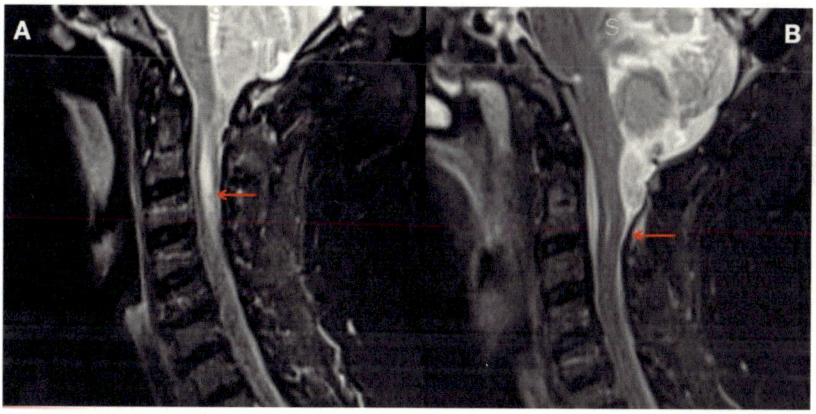

Figure 2.
A T2-weighted sagittal view of the cerebellum and cervical spine of our patient. In Panel A, we can see the compression of the cerebellum with a syrinx in the cervical spinal cord. Panel B shows decompression of the cerebellum with reduction in size of the syrinx in the spinal cord. The arrows point to the syrinx in these two images.

and returned to his normal function after 6 weeks. Eight months after surgery, he had a routine MRI with and without contrast that showed growth of three of his tumors. The patient was not symptomatic at the time. Given his history, the patient and his family elected to have these tumors treated with stereotactic radiosurgery. These tumors were treated with 12 Gy to a 50% isodose line (a relatively low dose of radiosurgery). Three months after this treatment, he developed gait instability, and MRI showed extensive edema associated with treated tumors. He was treated with dexamethasone (steroids) for 6 months. His symptoms resolved after several weeks of treatment. Unfortunately, we attempted to wean his steroids on three occasions with return of his symptoms. At this point, the patient was treated with bevacizumab infusion every 2 weeks. His swelling resolved after 4 cycles, and bevacizumab was discontinued. The patient is currently at his baseline and has continued follow-up in our multidisciplinary CNS clinic.

2. Literature review

Neurofibromatosis (NF) is a neurocutaneous syndrome characterized by the development of tumors of the central or peripheral nervous system including the brain, spinal cord, organs, skin, and bones [3]. Neurofibromatosis has three types: NF1, which is the most prevalent in 96% of the cases, NF2 in 3% of the cases, and schwannomatosis (SWN) in less than 1% of cases. NF1, or Von Recklinghausen's disease, causes a variety of clinical manifestations such as multiple flat, light-brown patches of skin pigment (café-au-lait spots), skin fold freckling, visible neurofibromas under the skin, and small nodules of the iris (Lisch nodules) [3]. NF1 gene located on 17q encodes a tumor suppressor protein called neurofibromin, a tumor suppressor protein that is produced in nerve cells, oligodendrocytes, and Schwann cells. A mutation in neurofibromin that renders it nonfunctional promotes the growth of neurofibromas throughout nerves in the entire body.

NF2 is an autosomal dominant multiple neoplasia syndrome that is a result of mutations in the NF2 suppressor gene, which is located on chromosome 22q [4]. The clinical diagnostic criteria have changed over time [5]. The current diagnostic criteria are described in **Table 1** [1, 2]. This gene encodes for the protein Merlin (moesin-ezrin-radixin-like protein) also known as Schwannomin [6]. Merlin is involved in the anchorage of the cytoskeleton to the cell membrane and is important for cell growth, protein translation, and cellular proliferation. Merlin blocks signaling caused by integrins and tyrosine receptor kinases at the membrane [7]. The absence of a normally functioning Merlin protein has been found to be associated with a predisposition to tumor formation [8]. This protein also negatively regulates Schwann cell production, and loss of this protein's functionality allows for Schwann cells to overproduce [7]. Various types of mutations, such as protein-truncating alterations (frameshift deletions/insertion and nonsense mutations), splice-site mutations, and missense mutations have been identified [9]. The milder type of NF2, Gardner type, has been found to be associated with missense mutations [10]. Nonsense/frameshift mutations produce a truncated protein and tend to be associated with a more severe phenotype, earlier onset, more rapid disease progression, and higher tumor burden with more spinal and intracranial tumors in addition to vestibular schwannomas [11].

Although many patients have symptoms before coming to medical attention, the average age of diagnosis of NF2 is 25 years [10]. Epidemiological studies place the incidence of NF2 between 1 in 33,000–40,000 live births, and there is no apparent difference in the proportion of men versus women who develop NF2 [10]. No prevalence has been described based on ethnicity. The actuarial survival after diagnosis is 15 years, and the average age of death is 36 years.

3. Tumors associated with NF2

Schwannomas are proliferations of neoplastic cells which show histologic, ultrastructural, and molecular similarities to the Schwann cells of the peripheral nervous system. They often arise at the glioma–Schwann cell junction within the internal auditory meatus and commonly arise from the superior vestibular nerve [10]. Vestibular schwannomas are the most common tumor in NF2 and are usually present bilaterally. Bilateral vestibular schwannomas are the distinctive feature of neurofibromatosis type 2 and are identified in 90–95% of patients [12]. This was the finding that established the diagnosis in our patient presented here (**Table 1**). Vestibular schwannomas clinically present as hearing loss progressing to deafness, dizziness and balance problems, tinnitus, facial nerve paralysis, and brainstem compression. Although more than 99% of vestibular schwannomas in NF2 are benign, they remain a substantial cause of morbidity because of their location [13]. Vestibular schwannomas rarely progress to malignancy, and sometimes unilateral vestibular schwannomas completely regress in size [14]. In the case presented here, the patient has partial hearing loss and functions well with hearing aids. His hearing is monitored annually, and he continues to do well. Trigeminal nerve schwannomas are the most commonly seen after vestibular, with oculomotor schwannomas following as the third most common schwannoma seen intracranially [10].

Meningiomas are the second most common tumor type in NF2, and the most common central nervous system tumor occurring throughout the central nervous system in 50–75% of individuals, often with multiple tumors [15]. Meningiomas are proliferations of neoplastic cells with histologic, ultrastructural, and immunophenotypic evidence of meningothelial cell differentiation. These proliferations can vary in histological appearances and genetic aberrations. Intracranial meningiomas are diagnosed in 45–58% of patients with NF2, and spinal meningiomas are diagnosed in approximately 20%. NF2-associated meningiomas occur most frequently in the supratentorial region in the frontal, parietal, and temporal regions as well as along the falx cerebri [16]. Although some meningiomas remain static and do not require active treatment, meningiomas associated with NF2 tend to be higher grade than sporadic tumors [5]. In the case discussed here, our patient has a predominance of meningiomas. Meningioma growth and associated swelling were the major cause of morbidity in this patient. Nearly all patients with NF2 develop meningiomas at some time throughout the progression of the syndrome. 50% of patients with NF2 present with schwannomas and meningiomas; 90% present with spine tumors in addition to schwannomas [10].

Ependymomas are proliferations of neoplastic cells with histologic, molecular, and ultrastructural similarities to the ependymal cells of the ventricles and spinal canal [16]. These tumors are diagnosed in approximately 33–53% of individuals with NF2, most commonly involving the posterior fossa and cervicomedullary region of the spine. Ependymomas associated with NF2 more often arise in patients who possess a truncating NF2 mutation, indicating that this tumor type is more associated with aggressive variants of NF2. Various spinal tumors may occur in patients with NF2 and can be found in the cervical, thoracic, and lumbar regions. Continued growth of spinal tumors causes loss of motion, numbness, tingling, and eventually paralysis [10].

Studies show that NF2 patients are frequently diagnosed with peripheral neuropathies [16]. Peripheral neuropathy in NF2 patients often presents as a mononeuropathy in children and as a polyneuropathy in adults. Nerve biopsies from patients with NF2 suggest that peripheral neuropathy results from local compression of nerves by Schwann cells tumors or non-mass-forming Schwann cell proliferations. Peripheral neuropathy can be difficult to treat and involves symptomatic control like neuropathic medication.

4. Patient presentation

Patients with NF2 can present with a variety of clinical manifestations. Ophthalmologic abnormalities are present in most patients, including cataracts (70–80%), retinal changes (20–44%), strabismus (12–50%), amblyopia (12%), optic nerve sheath meningiomas and other optic pathway tumors (10–27%), and extraocular movement abnormalities (10%). NF2 patients may also develop retinal hamartomas [16]. Cutaneous lesions are a frequent manifestation that patients present with NF2; however, cutaneous lesions are far more common with the NF1 subtype [16].

The cutaneous nodules associated with NF2 tend to present in a paler form and have more irregular margins in comparison to the lesions seen in NF1. There are three types of skin tumors that occur in NF2: NF2 plaques, nodular schwannomas, and neurofibromas. Approximately 70% of NF2 patients exhibit cutaneous lesions, and the most frequent type are “plaque-like” dermal plexiform schwannomas associated with slight pigmentation and increased hair growth. Subcutaneous nodular schwannomas that are associate with peripheral nerves are also present [16].

5. Patient management and treatment

The central goal of management of NF2 should be to maintain patient function and quality of life while managing tumor load. This can be extremely challenging. The literature shows strong evidence that these patients are best managed by a multidisciplinary team involving genetics, neurosurgery, otolaryngology, ophthalmology, neurology, radiology, pathology, and audiology [17]. Patients with NF2 at centers with this approach have better outcomes overall. We have embraced this multidisciplinary approach, and NF2 patients are followed in our Multidisciplinary CNS Tumor Clinic with these services available. In general, treatments for patients with NF2 can be divided into 4 major categories: conservative therapy, surgery, radiosurgery, and chemotherapy.

6. Conservative therapy

Despite the high prevalence of patients with multiple tumors, most meningiomas and spinal tumors are asymptomatic and are first discovered on MRI [10]. We recommend routine surveillance in all patients with NF2 whether or not they are symptomatic from their tumors. Patient visits should always include a complete physical examination and the appropriate imaging which usually includes a high-quality MRI of the brain and/or spine with and without contrast. MRIs are always compared to the previous MRIs for any detrimental changes. This comparison may be challenging in patients with multiple tumors in multiple locations (such as the patient presented here). A dedicated neuroradiologist is essential in these cases. The frequency of visits and imaging may vary from 4 months to annually based on clinical parameters. Patients with vestibular schwannomas require regular audiology evaluations, and patients with tumors affecting the optic pathway require regular vision evaluations. At our center, this is performed by a neuro-ophthalmologist. The patient discussed here was found to have asymptotic tumor growth during a routine surveillance visit. Such care allows tumors to be treated before they can grow to larger sizes.

7. Surgery

Surgery is often the treatment of choice when an NF2 patient has a tumor that is actively growing. Growing meningiomas may result in increased intracranial pressure, intractable headaches, hydrocephalus, and seizure disorders [10]. The patient presented here had symptoms from direct cerebral and cerebellar compression as well as hydrocephalus. In the case of this patient, surgery was necessary, and the patient derived great benefit from this intervention. Meningiomas involving the skull base may be much more difficult to remove and have a higher risk of postoperative neurological morbidity. Spinal meningiomas and schwannomas can cause symptomatic compression and often require surgery. The difficulty of removing these tumors depends on tumor size and location. Ependymomas rarely require removal. However, when spinal ependymomas are removed, they may also be challenging and require an experienced team. Vestibular schwannomas should be surgically addressed when they are growing because they can cause brainstem compression, hearing loss, and facial paralysis. We firmly believe that these tumors should be operated at centers that have multidisciplinary teams that manage a high volume of patients.

The patient presented here also had an additional surgery for decompression of an acquired Chiari malformation with associated syrinx, or expanded space within the spinal cord. A Chiari malformation is defined as the caudal displacement of the cerebellar tonsils below the level of the foramen magnum [18]. Syringomyelia, or the presence of a syrinx, can present in 30–70% of cases and can cause neurological deficits [19]. The cause of this problem is the lack of flow across the foramen magnum, and first-line treatment involves restoring this flow surgically. Adequate decompression with restoration of flow leads to resolution of the syrinx with abatement of symptoms. In this case, our patient presented with difficulty with balance and developed bilateral hand weakness; both are classical symptoms of cervical syrinx. In this case, the patient had known posterior fossa crowding that improved after decompression. We attribute his development of a syrinx to both scarring after surgery, which can decrease the flow of CSF across the foramen magnum, and residual compression caused by other tumors in his posterior fossa that were not addressed by his previous surgery. As expected, surgical decompression of the posterior fossa, cervical laminectomies, and duroplasty restored the flow of CSF from his posterior fossa to the spinal canal and resulted in deflation of his syrinx and complete resolution of his symptoms. Although this is not a problem that is unique to patients with NF2 or meningiomas, this case is instructive in the management of acquired Chiari malformation and the management of associated syrinx.

8. Radiosurgery

Stereotactic radiosurgery (SRS), or radiosurgery, is a treatment of tumors and other lesions using well-collimated, multiple small beams of ionizing radiation to treat a target, while reducing toxic exposure to surrounding tissues. SRS has been shown to be a safe and effective treatment for vestibular schwannomas and meningiomas in patients who do not have NF2 [20–22]. A recent study has shown that this is also the case in patients with NF2 [23]. These authors showed that in 18 patients with 120 convexity meningiomas, radiosurgery achieved a 99.1% tumor control rate with only a 0.8% risk of radiation-induced adverse events. The tumor volume ranged from 0.10 to 21.3 cm^3 (median 0.66 cm^3), with a median marginal dose range of 12–25 Gy (median 12 Gy) in this study. These results show that radiosurgery was safe and effective overall. Our patient experienced radiation-induced edema that had a protracted course after treatment with radiosurgery. The tumors treated in our patient were 5.9, 11.5, and 26.1 cm^3 and were all treated with 12 Gy to the 50% isodose line. The radiation doses between tumors were negligible. Given that our patient had swelling associated with even the smallest tumor treated, we suspect that this is an idiosyncratic outcome that we cannot attribute to radiation dose or tumor size.

9. Chemotherapy

There are established chemotherapy treatments for NF2. Vascular endothelial growth factor (VEGF)-A is important in the growth of schwannomas [24, 25]. Studies have shown tumor shrinkage and hearing improvement after patients begin treatment with bevacizumab (a monoclonal antibody against VEGF-A) [25–29]. There are a number of ongoing phase II clinical trials looking at this drug as a possible treatment. There are ongoing phase II clinical trials evaluating other agents including Icotinib, Axitinib, everolimus, Crizotinib, Brigatinib, and Selumetinib [3]. There is no current chemotherapy for meningiomas. The current data for the treatment of meningiomas with bevacizumab are mixed at best [30–34]. Our patient was placed on bevacizumab to treat his cerebral edema. Although this was quite effective in reducing the swelling associated with his tumor, there was no notable changes in the size of either of his vestibular schwannomas or meningiomas secondary to bevacizumab.

10. Conclusion

In our case report, we detail the care of one of our patients with NF2. We have used this case to emphasize the challenges involved in the care of these patients. This patient has done well overall secondary to the care provided to him by all of his providers. We have also reviewed the literature of NF2 and other conditions affecting his care. Our goal with this description and review of the literature is to better elucidate the needs of these patients and the issues involved in providing care for patients with NF2.

Author details

Tayler D. Payton[1] and Marcus L. Ware[2]*

1 Louisiana State University School of Medicine, New Orleans, Louisiana, United States

2 Department of Oncology Neurosurgery, Ochsner Medical Center, New Orleans, Louisiana, USA

*Address all correspondence to: marcusware@gmail.com

IntechOpen

© 2023 The Author(s). Licensee IntechOpen. This chapter is distributed under the terms of the Creative Commons Attribution License (http://creativecommons.org/licenses/by/3.0), which permits unrestricted use, distribution, and reproduction in any medium, provided the original work is properly cited.

References

[1] Smith MJ et al. Revisiting neurofibromatosis type 2 diagnostic criteria to exclude LZTR1-related schwannomatosis. Neurology. 2017;**88**(1):87-92

[2] Evans DG et al. Identifying the deficiencies of current diagnostic criteria for neurofibromatosis 2 using databases of 2777 individuals with molecular testing. Genetics in Medicine. 2019;**21**(7):1525-1533

[3] Tamura R. Current understanding of Neurofibromatosis type 1, 2, and Schwannomatosis. International Journal of Molecular Sciences. 2021;**22**(11):1-17

[4] Asthagiri AR et al. Neurofibromatosis type 2. Lancet. 2009;**373**(9679):1974-1986

[5] Bachir S et al. Neurofibromatosis type 2 (NF2) and the implications for vestibular Schwannoma and meningioma pathogenesis. International Journal of Molecular Sciences. 2021;**22**(2):1-21

[6] Lutchman M, Rouleau GA. The neurofibromatosis type 2 gene product, schwannomin, suppresses growth of NIH 3T3 cells. Cancer Research. 1995;**55**(11):2270-2274

[7] Obremski VJ, Hall AM, Fernandez-Valle C. Merlin, the neurofibromatosis type 2 gene product, and beta1 integrin associate in isolated and differentiating Schwann cells. Journal of Neurobiology. 1998;**37**(4):487-501

[8] Lee S et al. The role of Merlin/NF2 loss in meningioma biology. Cancers (Basel). 2019;**11**(11):1-25

[9] Petrilli AM, Fernandez-Valle C. Role of Merlin/NF2 inactivation in tumor biology. Oncogene. 2016;**35**(5):537-548

[10] Slattery WH. Neurofibromatosis type 2. Otolaryngologic Clinics of North America. 2015;**48**(3):443-460

[11] Dispenza F, Martines F. Vestibular Schwannoma : Pathophysiology, Diagnosis and Treatment. Rare Disorders Research Progress. New York: Nova Science Publishers, Inc; 2020. p. 243

[12] Fisher LM et al. Concordance of bilateral vestibular schwannoma growth and hearing changes in neurofibromatosis 2: Neurofibromatosis 2 natural history consortium. Otology & Neurotology. 2009;**30**(6):835-841

[13] Slattery WH 3rd et al. Vestibular schwannoma growth rates in neurofibromatosis type 2 natural history consortium subjects. Otology & Neurotology. 2004;**25**(5):811-817

[14] Merker VL et al. Health-related quality of life of individuals with Neurofibromatosis type 2: Results from the NF2 natural history study. Otology & Neurotology. 2016;**37**(5):574-579

[15] Eckstein O et al. Multiple meningiomas in brain and lung due to acquired mutation of the NF2 gene. Neurology. 2004;**62**(10):1904-1905

[16] Coy S et al. An update on the CNS manifestations of neurofibromatosis type 2. Acta Neuropathologica. 2020;**139**(4):643-665

[17] Lloyd SK, Evans DG. Neurofibromatosis type 2 (NF2): Diagnosis and management. Handbook of Clinical Neurology. 2013;**115**:957-967

[18] Wang J et al. Acquired Chiari malformation and Syringomyelia secondary to space-occupying lesions: A systematic review. World Neurosurgery. 2017;**98**:800-808

[19] Greenberg MS. Greenberg's Handbook of Neurosurgery. 10th ed. New York: Thieme; 2023

[20] Lippitz BE et al. Ten-year follow-up after gamma knife radiosurgery of meningioma and review of the literature. Acta Neurochirurgica. 2020;**162**(9):2183-2196

[21] Jakubeit T et al. Single-fraction stereotactic radiosurgery versus microsurgical resection for the treatment of vestibular schwannoma: A systematic review and meta-analysis. Systematic Reviews. 2022;**11**(1):265

[22] Jayaprakash S, Pendse AM, Deshpande S. Significance of dosimetric parameters in patients undergoing gamma knife radiosurgery for vestibular Schwannoma. Journal of Medical Physics. 2022;**47**(2):206-211

[23] Ruiz-Garcia H et al. Convexity Meningiomas in patients with Neurofibromatosis type 2: Long-term outcomes after gamma knife radiosurgery. World Neurosurgery. 2021;**146**:e678-e684

[24] Caye-Thomasen P et al. VEGF and VEGF receptor-1 concentration in vestibular schwannoma homogenates correlates to tumor growth rate. Otology & Neurotology. 2005;**26**(1):98-101

[25] Komotar RJ et al. The role of bevacizumab in hearing preservation and tumor volume control in patients with vestibular schwannomas. Neurosurgery. 2009;**65**(6):N12

[26] Eminowicz GK et al. Bevacizumab treatment for vestibular schwannomas in neurofibromatosis type two: Report of two cases, including responses after prior gamma knife and vascular endothelial growth factor inhibition therapy. The Journal of Laryngology and Otology. 2012;**126**(1):79-82

[27] Blakeley J et al. Clinical response to bevacizumab in schwannomatosis. Neurology. 2014;**83**(21):1986-1987

[28] Alanin MC et al. The effect of bevacizumab on vestibular schwannoma tumour size and hearing in patients with neurofibromatosis type 2. European Archives of Oto-Rhino-Laryngology. 2015;**272**(12):3627-3633

[29] Karajannis MA et al. Sustained imaging response and hearing preservation with low-dose bevacizumab in sporadic vestibular schwannoma. Neuro-Oncology. 2019;**21**(6):822-824

[30] Shih KC et al. A phase II trial of bevacizumab and everolimus as treatment for patients with refractory, progressive intracranial meningioma. Journal of Neuro-Oncology. 2016;**129**(2):281-288

[31] Dasanu CA et al. Bevacizumab in refractory higher-grade and atypical meningioma: The current state of affairs. Expert Opinion on Biological Therapy. 2019;**19**(2):99-104

[32] Mathew Thomas V, Bindal P, Vredenburgh JJ. Everolimus and bevacizumab in the Management of Recurrent, progressive intracranial NF2 mutated meningioma. Case Report Oncologia. 2019;**12**(1):126-130

[33] Scerrati A et al. The controversial role of bevacizumab in the treatment of patients with intracranial meningioma: A comprehensive literature review. Expert Review of Anticancer Therapy. 2020;**20**(3):197-203

[34] Kumthekar P et al. A multi-institutional phase II trial of bevacizumab for recurrent and refractory meningioma. Neurooncological Advances. 2022;**4**(1):vdac123

Section 3

Treatment and Management of Neurofibromatosis

Chapter 3

Immunotherapy Strategies for NF2-Associated Tumors

Shyam Patel, Thomas C. Chen and Frances E. Chow

Abstract

Considering the limited benefit of current therapies for NF2-associated tumors, immunotherapy prevails as a promising treatment strategy with the potential to selectively eliminate tumor cells. This chapter focuses on the concepts of cancer immunotherapy, specific challenges unique to nervous system tumors, and current preclinical studies and clinical trials. We highlight several promising advances which may help to overcome the unmet therapeutic need in NF2-associated tumors.

Keywords: immunotherapy, emerging therapy, clinical trials, NF2-associated tumors, immunotherapy strategies

1. Introduction

Neurofibromatosis type 2 (NF2) is characterized by the development of nervous system tumors including vestibular schwannomas, meningiomas, and ependymomas [1–3]. Although these tumors are typically histologically benign, they may exhibit aggressive growth, cause devastating neurological disability, and lead to complications that result in early mortality [4, 5]. Current treatments for NF2 associated tumors involve multidisciplinary collaborations and include surgical resection, possible radiation, and chemotherapy—all of which are non-curative and are associated with the risk of permanent hearing loss or future development of malignancy [6, 7]. The identification of two-hit alterations to the NF2 gene on chromosome 22q12 [8, 9] and subsequent aberrations in the merlin and PI3k/Akt/mTOR pathways have led to extensive investigations into targeted therapies, yet none have demonstrated significant benefit to garner approval [10–20]. Therefore, a significant unmet need exists in the management of NF2 associated tumors.

Immunotherapy prevails as an appealing treatment strategy due to its potential to generate tumor-specific responses to selectively eliminate tumor cells. Since 2014, growing success in liquid and solid tumors has resulted in over 50 separate United States Food and Drug Administration approvals for immunotherapies [21]. Notable exceptions to the list of indications are central and peripheral nervous system tumors. This chapter focuses on the underpinning principles of immunotherapy, specific challenges unique to nervous system tumors, and promising emerging advances which may overcome the unmet therapeutic need in NF2 associated tumors.

2. Immunotherapy strategies

The immune system recognizes deviations from natural homeostasis as dangerous and employs the innate and adaptive immune systems to protect the body from "non-self" such as bacteria, viruses, and cancer. While innate immunity drives rapid responses through evolutionarily conserved mechanisms, adaptive immunity develops over days and is honed against specific antigens. In applying this concept to cancer immunology, it is possible to leverage each of the key executors—the cancer cell, antigen presenting cell, and effector T cell—as an immunotherapeutic strategy (**Figure 1**).

2.1 Leveraging tumor: cancer vaccines and oncolytic viruses

Direct targeting of the tumor cell has been attempted through methods such as cancer vaccines and oncolytic viruses.

Vaccines are designed to prime the immune system to induce a tumor-directed response. Crucial to this mechanism is the identification of a pre-identified tumor specific antigen. Cautionary tales in tumor antigen escape were identified through experience in glioblastoma with rindopepimut (CDX-110), an epidermal growth

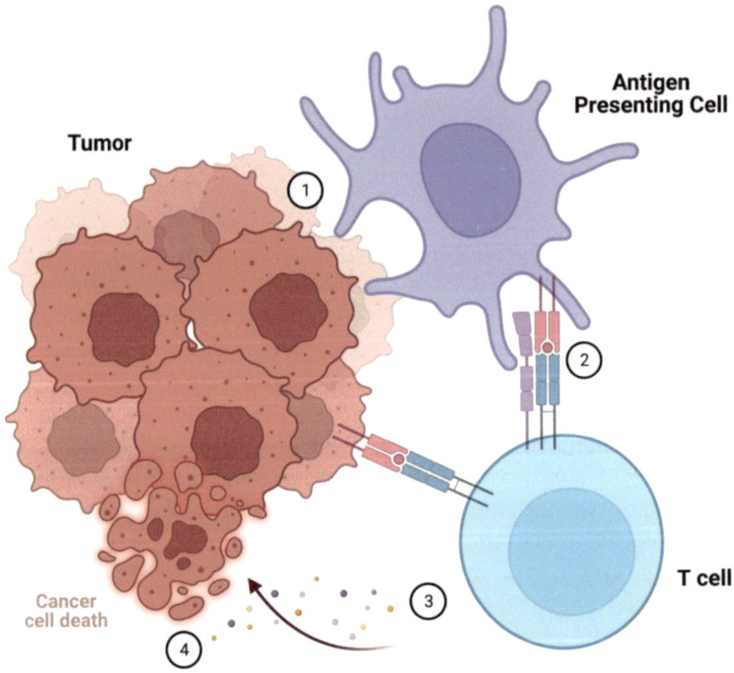

Figure 1.
*Cancer immunology and principles of immunotherapy. (1) Tumor cells undergo phagocytosis by an antigen presenting cell (APC). (2) The APC presents tumor associated antigens on an MHC molecule to a naïve T cell. Dendritic cells have the most effective antigen presentation and T cell activation. Macrophages are subtyped into M1 anti-tumor and M2 pro-tumor/anti-inflammatory. Natural killer cells are part of the innate immune system and are capable of both antigen presentation and T cell activation. (3) T cell activation occurs when the appropriate T cell receptor (TCR) pairs with a matching tumor-associated antigen. Additional costimulatory signals such as B7-CD28 and cytokines are necessary to guide the differentiation and expansion of effector cells into cytotoxic T cells, helper T cells, regulatory T cells, and B cells. Each of these effector cells have unique markers and functions (**Table 1**). (4) The cytotoxic T cell eliminates the cancer cell in a process involving perforins, granzymes, and lysozymes.*

Cell type	Markers	Function
Cytotoxic T cell	TCR, CD8+	Kill cells
Helper T cell	TCR, CD4+	Enhance immune function
Regulatory T cell	TCR, CD4+	Dampen immune function
B cell	BCR	Antibody production

Table 1.
Effector cell types.

factor receptor variant III (EGFRvIII) "vaccine" composed of EGFRvIII conjugated to the potent immunogenic substance KLH. Rindopepimut effectively activated humoral immunity through the endogenous formation of EGFRvIII antibodies. In a series of early phase clinical trials in recurrent glioblastoma, rindopepimut demonstrated improvement in overall survival [22–25]. However, the phase 3 study was terminated early for futility, as survival was similar in the experimental and control arms [26]. Although 84% of tumors that originally expressed EGFRvIII lost expression at recurrence, this phenomenon of antigen escape was observed in both the control and treatment arms—thereby challenging the notion that EGFRvIII targeting therapies were solely responsible for the outgrowth of EGFRvIII-deficient glioblastoma cells.

The challenge with cancer vaccines remains difficulty in identifying a tumor-associated antigen and the intrinsic evolution of antigens over time through antigen escape. However, a potential alternative to vaccines based on pre-identified high quality endogenous neoantigens is through in-situ introduction of tumor-associated antigens via oncolytic viruses.

Oncolytic viruses are engineered to selectively infect cancer cells, leading to cell death and endogenous release of tumor antigens to promote a secondary immune response. An example of an oncolytic virus is the recombinant nonpathogenic polio-rhinovirus chimera, which infects malignant cells via CD155 receptor and causes tumor cell death. This releases tumor antigens into the microenvironment, attracting immune cells which then are sub-lethally infected by the virus to create a sustained pro-inflammatory cytokine response [27]. Additional viruses modified for oncolytic purposes include herpes, adeno, reo, vaccinia, measles, newcastle, and parvovirus [28].

2.2 Leveraging antigen presenting cells: dendritic cell vaccines, macrophages, natural killer cells

Dendritic cells represent the most effective antigen presenting cell in phagocytosing cancer cells and training T cells. Dendritic cell vaccines have been a mainstay of immunotherapy through the leukapheresis, *ex vivo* loading or pulsing with various antigen sources (including peptides, DNA, RNA, liposomes), and then delivery of dendritic cells intradermally as a "vaccine" administered to the patient. The concept of dendritic cell vaccines has been explored in several groups, with recent promise demonstrated in newly diagnosed glioblastoma [29].

Macrophages make up the predominant immune infiltrate within intracranial tumors. For example, in vestibular schwannomas, macrophages—rather than Schwann cells—constitute up to 70% of proliferating cells [30]. Macrophages confer both anti-tumor (M1) and pro-tumor (M2) properties. Tumor-associated macrophage markers remain under investigation, but M1 macrophages (iNOS+, CD86+,

CD80+, HLA-DR+) are classically tumor-resistant in the setting of phagocytotic and antitumor inflammatory signatures. Alternatively, M2 macrophages (CD206+, CD204+, CD163+) promote immunosuppression, angiogenesis, and neovascularization [31]. The unique balance of immune-stimulating and immunosuppressive properties marks macrophages as an ideal candidate for immune modulation and directed polarization.

Natural killer (NK) cells represent 5–15% of circulating lymphocytes [32]. As members of the innate immune system, they are not limited by MHC restriction and do not require priming. To date, NK cells have encountered minimal issues with cytokine release syndrome (as with CAR T cells) and maintain antigen specificity such as for antibody-mediated cell engagers. NK cells therefore serve as appealing targets of immunotherapy.

2.3 Leveraging effector cytotoxic T cells: adoptive transfer, CAR T cells, checkpoint inhibitors, BITE therapies

T cells serve as the end effector to trigger tumor cytotoxicity through lysozymes, granzymes, and perforins. Potential mechanisms of T cell manipulation include adoptive transfer of genetically engineered CAR T cells, reversal of T cell exhaustion through checkpoint inhibitors, and localization of T cells to targets through bispecific T cell engagers (BITEs).

Adoptive transfer precipitates T cell activation by enlisting T cells through harvesting of autologous T cells, which are trained and expanded ex vivo against tumor, and transferred back to patients. However, there is significant difficulty in generating large numbers of functional tumor-specific T cells.

Out of this need arose the concept of CAR T cells, which are genetically modified T cells expressing chimeric antigen receptors (CARs). Such engineered CARs are chimeric because they combine both antigen-binding and T-cell activating functions into a single receptor (**Figure 2**). CARs are thereby programmed to recognize antigen without the need for MHC presentation or costimulatory signals to activate proliferation or clonal expansion in situ. Additional CAR modifications include *bispecific* CARs that target multiple tumor-associated antigens to minimize off-tumor effects or mitigate antigen escape; *masked* CARs with tumor-expressed proteases capable of cleaving linkers to scFvs of CARs for selective activation specifically by tumor cells; and *switchable* CARs to target peptide neo-epitopes present on a tumor-associated antigen-binding antibody (rather than the tumor cell) [33].

In a case report from a phase 1 clinical trial for IL13Ra2 CAR T, a patient with recurrent multifocal intracranial glioblastoma underwent resection and direct intratumoral infusion with CAR T cells with local control. However, he subsequently developed continued progression of non-resected areas and developed leptomeningeal spread with spinal metastases. Additional intraventricular infusions of CAR T cells via a rickham reservoir led to dramatic clinical and radiographic response that lasted 7.5 months; however his disease ultimately recurred [34]. CAR T cells have thus far had limited efficacy in brain tumors due to antigen escape, limited T cell persistence, exhaustion, and adequate delivery to the tumor.

An effective mechanism of crosslinking T cells to their target is through bispecific T cell engagers (BITEs). BITEs are antibody constructs comprised of a CD3 antigen binding segment and a tumor-antigen binding segment.

All T cells, including engineered CAR T cells, demonstrate limited persistence due to exhaustion over time. T cell expression of CTLA-4 and PD-1, as well as engagement

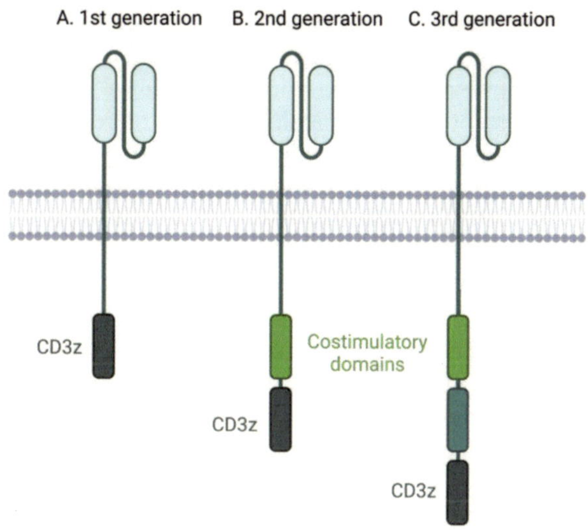

Figure 2.
CAR T cells of 1st generation, 2nd generation, 3rd generation. (A) 1st generation CARs exhibit single chain variable fragment to target a tumor antigen moiety and are limited by poor persistence. (B) 2nd generation CARs are supplemented by the presence of a co-stimulatory domain and are associated with increased toxicity. (C) 3rd generation CARs have both co-stimulatory domains.

with PD-L1, deactivates T cells and triggers apoptosis. Checkpoint blockade with ipilimumab, nivolumab, atezolizumab, or pembrolizumab inhibits these inhibitory signals, thereby re-activating exhausted T cells. Checkpoint inhibitors are of interest because they are off the shelf; however, they have had limited benefit as a monotherapy in nervous system tumors. There remains significant promise in the use of checkpoint inhibitors (and other checkpoints such as IDO1 and TIM3) neoadjuvant to surgery [35, 36], with radiation [37], or in combination with other immune modulating therapies.

3. Unique challenges to immunotherapy

Despite the elegant simplicity of the immune system, many intrinsic and extrinsic obstacles pose therapeutic challenges to immunotherapy via immune escape, immune privilege, low tumor antigenicity, and a cold tumor microenvironment. Immunotherapy aims to counteract each of these intrinsic hurdles and tumor evasion techniques.

3.1 Cancer immune escape

Cancer immune escape is based upon the theory of immune surveillance, in which the immune system recognizes and destroys transformed cells before they give rise to detectable tumors. However, the building burden of genetic instability and immune pressure leads to immune escape and ultimately tumor progression.

3.2 Immune privilege and the blood-brain barrier

Historically, the central nervous system (CNS) has been considered an immune privileged organ due to an intact blood brain barrier and absence of a typical lymphatic system. Early studies in rabbits demonstrated that allogeneic skin grafts placed on different organs of the body were rapidly rejected, but skin grafts placed on the brain escaped rejection [38]. However, this assumption of immune privilege has been challenged considering recent evidence for CNS lymphatics, or glymphatics [39–41]. Evidence for CNS lymphatics was based on observations that radiolabeled polyethylene glycol and albumin injected in the brain could be detected in the cervical lymphatics and along the olfactory nerve [42–46]. Further work described an additional route for the egress of soluble antigen via perivenous and periarterial structures [39, 40].

Therefore, the brain is not as immunologically privileged as once thought. But it continues to hold true that the blood-brain barrier limits the traversing of molecules, recombinant proteins, or gene-based medicines that are larger than 50 Da. Poor penetration across the blood-brain barrier occurs with approximately 98% of small molecule drugs and nearly all large molecules. Most chemotherapies, targeted therapies, and drug-antibody conjugates unfortunately do not cross the blood-brain barrier [47, 48].

3.3 Low tumor antigenicity

A second mechanism of immune escape is inherent to the tumor itself. Nervous system tumors have low antigenicity, making it difficult for the immune system to recognize the tumor as non-self to generate an immune response. Tumor-associated antigens may be identified through genetic, biochemical, and predictive computational approaches [49].

3.3.1 Low tumor mutational burden

The success of immunotherapy in melanoma and NSCLC is in part due to the high tumor mutational burden from UV- and smoking-related DNA damage. A high tumor mutational load provides a high availability of neoantigens, which are easily recognized by the patrolling immune system to induce an antitumor immune response [50–53]. However in glioblastoma, fewer than 4% of glioblastomas have an inherent high tumor mutational burden, as the median tumor mutational burden is 4 [54].

3.3.2 Rarity of common tumor-specific antigens

As an alternative to overall mutational load, antigens of high tumoral specificity may serve as an optimal target for the immune system. Across patients there unfortunately exists a low number of shared common mutations in NF2 associated tumors. Additionally, in gliomas there is significant heterogeneity within a single tumor, as a tumor-associated antigen is not necessarily expressed on every cell across a tumor. Furthermore, as observed in the example of the tumor-specific antigen EGFRvIII, expression of tumor antigens varies not only with location, but also with time. Serial evaluation of tumors demonstrates transformation over time, such as with the loss of the tumor-associated antigen EGFRvIII in glioblastoma [26], thereby contributing to immune escape.

3.4 Cold tumor microenvironment

Gliomas notoriously create a highly immunosuppressive microenvironment characterized by few functional antigen presenting cells, in addition to abundant immunosuppressive APCs and regulatory T cells [55]. We continue to learn more about the abundant monocytic and dendritic cell populations which predominate the bulk of tumor infiltrating immune cells [56–58]. Brain tumors such as glioblastoma are therefore considered immunologically "cold."

4. Vestibular schwannomas

4.1 Background

Over the past several decades, significant research has been conducted to understand the underlying mechanisms of vestibular schwannoma development and to identify effective treatments for these tumors. It has been long recognized that regions of inflammatory cells penetrate vestibular schwannomas (Antoni B regions) [59]. Serum and tumor extracts from patients with vestibular schwannomas overexpress immunogenic mediators including IL-1B, IL-6, TNF-a, ICAM-1, and CXCR4 [60–67]. Fast-growing vestibular schwannomas express elevated IL-34 and M-CSF, which may be responsible for chemotaxis of tumor associated macrophages [68] and higher levels of inflammation correlating with longer duration of symptoms [69].

More recent work has explored the role of inflammation [30] and identification of precise tumor infiltrating immune populations in vestibular schwannomas [70, 71]. CD163+ tumor-associated macrophages (M2) are associated with the volumetric growth of vestibular schwannomas [72] and shorter progression-free survival [73–76]. Regulatory T cells (CD4+, CD25+, FOXP3+) suppress tumor-specific immunity [77] and are more prominent in progressive vestibular schwannomas [78, 79]. Progressive vestibular schwannomas in patients demonstrate increased expression of PD-L1 and other checkpoints such as TIM-3 [80], potentially implicating a mechanism of PD-L1 mediated immune evasion [81, 82].

4.2 Immunotherapy strategies

4.2.1 Checkpoint inhibitor

Preclinical and clinical investigations have explored the potential role of checkpoint inhibitors in the management of vestibular schwannomas. Mouse models treated with PD-1 blockade successfully demonstrated reduction in schwannoma size, underscoring the potential therapeutic effect of checkpoint inhibitors in vestibular schwannomas [83].

4.2.2 Oncolytic bacteria

A recent preclinical study employed the bacterial cancer theory to demonstrate the effectiveness of intratumoral injections of bacteria within hypoxic areas of angiogenic tumors, thereby triggering lysis of tumor cells and antitumor responses [84] such as shift of macrophages from M2 (pro-tumor) to M1 (anti-tumor) subtypes [85, 86]. In human xenograft and mouse syngeneic models, a highly attenuated strain of *Salmonella typhimurium* (VNP00002) was capable of inducing cytokine and effector cell profiles toward enhanced innate and adaptive immune responses to control the growth of intrasciatic benign schwannomas [87]. The mechanism is consistent with a vaccination-based immunotherapy and supports further evaluation in NF2 vestibular schwannomas.

4.3 Future directions

These preclinical results provide important evidence to support the potential role of immunotherapy in the treatment of NF2-associated vestibular schwannomas. Clinical trials are needed to fully understand the safety and efficacy of this approach and to determine the optimal treatment regimen for patients with this condition.

5. Meningiomas

5.1 Background

An understanding of the intricate interaction between meningiomas and the immune system offers opportunities for immunotherapy-based treatments. Within meningiomas, up to one quarter of all cells are macrophages [88–91]. Macrophages make up the largest fraction of immune infiltrates (up to 80%) [89] and are predominantly the immunosuppressive M2 phenotype [92]. High grade meningiomas and recurrent meningiomas harbor a higher proportion of M2 macrophages [88, 93], and M2 macrophages are independently associated with worse prognosis [94]. Other immune infiltrates include T cells and B cells [95]. Although the degree of Treg infiltration has not yet been demonstrated as an independent prognostic factor, grade 3 meningiomas have increased penetration of Tregs, supporting the potential role of immunosuppression in developing resistance and immune escape [96]. Further contribution to an immunosuppressive response in meningiomas is the high expression of several checkpoint molecules including NY-ESO-1, PC-L1, PD-L2, B7-H3, and CTLA-4 [96–100], which have been associated with tumor recurrence, progression, and worse prognosis [99].

5.2 Immunotherapy strategies

5.2.1 Interferon-alpha

The initial use of immune modulating therapies in meningiomas employed the cytokine interferon-alpha (IFN-a). A pilot study in both low and high grade meningiomas demonstrated that treatment with IFN-a demonstrated a slight regression or stable disease lasting from 6 to 14 months (n = 6) [101]. An additional phase 2 trial in grade 1 meningiomas demonstrated a 6-month progression free survival (PFS-6) of 54% and a median progression free survival (mPFS) of 7 months [102]. However, a retrospective cohort study in high grade meningiomas demonstrated a limited PFS-6 of only 17% and mPFS of 3 months [103]. These studies served as proof-of-concept in the potential role of immune modulation for meningiomas.

5.2.2 Checkpoint inhibitors

In a recent phase 2 trial evaluating the efficacy of pembrolizumab in sporadic recurrent grade 2 and 3 meningiomas (n = 24), PFS-6 was 0.48 (90% CI: 0.31–0.66) and mPFS reached 7.6 months (90% CI: 3.4–12.9 months). The adverse event profile matched that of other PD-1 inhibitor studies, including fatigue, pruritis, and 20% experienced CTCAE grade 3 or higher adverse events [104]. Another recent phase 2 trial evaluating the efficacy of nivolumab in recurrent grade 2 and 3 meningiomas (n = 25) demonstrated PFS-6 of 42.4% (95% CI: 22.8–60.7) and median overall survival of 30.9 months (95% CI: 17.6-NA). The investigators concluded that a subset of patients benefitted from therapy but overall, the study did not meet its predefined endpoint [105]. Although these studies were not strictly for NF2 associated meningiomas, the results warrant further investigation, particularly in a dedicated NF2 population.

5.2.3 Adoptive transfer

We currently await results from a recently-completed phase 2 trial which evaluated anti-NY-ESO1 T cell receptor-gene engineered lymphocytes [106]. In this study, 11 patients with NY-ESO1-expressing tumors (melanoma, meningioma, breast cancer, non-small cell lung cancer, and hepatocellular cancer) were treated with T cells that had undergone TCR-engineering via retroviral transfection. The patients completed lymphodepletion with cyclophosphamide and fludarabine prior to infusion of the modified T cells with enhancement by aldesleukin. If beneficial, this study may support prior preclinical data in targeting NY-ESO-1 as an immunotherapeutic strategy for the treatment of meningiomas [107].

5.3 Future directions

These clinical trials provide evidence of the potential of immunotherapy as a treatment option for meningiomas. However, it is important to note that these studies are preliminary and that more research is needed to determine the best approach for incorporating immunotherapy into the treatment of NF2-associated meningiomas.

6. Ependymomas

6.1 Background

Genomic analysis has demonstrated that ependymomas are molecularly distinct from gliomas such as glioblastoma. However, as a subtype of gliomas, significant interest and investigation is ongoing in the ependymoma tumor microenvironment and potential immunotherapy targets. Qualitative analysis of tumor-infiltrating immune populations reveals that increased cytotoxic T cells (CD8+), a high ratio of CD4+/CD8+ cells, and increased number of IDO+ cells (dendritic cells) are associated with favorable prognosis. Alternatively, elevated FOXP3+ Tregs, CD68+ TAMs, and M2 polarization (high ratio of CD163/AIF1+ cells) are associated with poor prognosis [108].

Ependymomas express a subset of unique tumor-associated antigens which may serve as potential targets for vaccine or oncolytic therapies due to their selective overexpression in tumor compared to normal brain tissue, including EphA2, IL-13Ra2, Survivin, and WT1 [109, 110]. Response to bevacizumab in NF2 associated ependymomas [111, 112] suggests that VEGF may serve as another target antigen for further immunotherapy development. This builds upon prior work demonstrating that more significant immune responses may correlate with improved survival [113].

6.2 Immunotherapy strategies

6.2.1 Peptide vaccine

There is an ongoing phase 1 trial of the SurVaxM vaccine in children with progressive or relapsed ependymoma, medulloblastoma, high grade glioma or newly diagnosed diffuse intrinsic pontine glioma (NCT04978727) [114]. The SurVaxM vaccine targets Survivin, a protein that stabilizes microtubules during spindle formation and whose high expression in several malignancies including ependymomas is associated with unfavorable prognosis [115]. The vaccine employs several strategies to create an antitumor effect, including through the incorporation and enhanced binding of multiple MHC class I epitopes, cytokine support, and antibody-mediated cell killing. SurVaxM has completed a phase 2 trial in newly diagnosed glioblastoma, with no serious adverse events [116].

Under investigation for children with recurrent ependymoma is an additional tumor antigen peptide-mediated vaccine. In this phase 1 trial, HLA-A2 restricted synthetic tumor antigens will be administered in combination with the immunoadjuvant imiquimod to stimulate an immune response (NCT01795313) [117]. We eagerly await results from these trials.

6.2.2 Oncolytic virus

The ongoing phase 1 trial of oncolytic HSV-1 G207 in combination with single dose radiation for children with recurrent or refractory cerebellar brain tumors seeks to use an engineered herpes simplex virus-1 to selectively replicate in and kill tumor cells (NCT03911388) [118]. While several past and ongoing oncolytic HSV brain tumor trials have been completed, therapeutic resistance has remained a challenge in relation to intratumoral delivery of the viral vector, the tumor microenvironment, and failure of the host's immune response [119].

6.2.3 CAR T cell therapy

Adoptive transfer with CAR T cells is an active area of investigation for ependymomas. Microarray analysis of pediatric ependymomas identify the human epidermal growth factor receptor 2 (HER2) as a potential tumor-associated antigen target, with preclinical experiments confirming antigen recognition [120]. There is an ongoing phase 1 trial of HER2 specific CAR T cells in children with recurrent or refractory ependymomas (NCT04903080) [121]. Additionally, there is an ongoing phase 1 trial of IL-13Ra2 CAR T cells in adults with ependymoma, leptomeningeal glioblastoma, or medulloblastoma (NCT04903080) [122]. Up to 67% of ependymoma cells express IL-13Ra2, which is associated with poor prognosis [123]. Early benefit with IL-13Ra2 CAR T cells in refractory glioblastoma [34] supports its use as a feasible therapy in ependymomas.

However, considering lessons learned from glioblastoma, concerns for an immunosuppressive microenvironment and tumor heterogeneity may limit the effectiveness of single-target CAR T therapies in ependymomas [124]. Tandem CAR T cells targeting more than 1 tumor-associated antigen may help to mitigate tumor antigen escape [125].

6.2.4 Checkpoint inhibitor

An ongoing phase 1 trial is evaluating the safety and preliminary efficacy of pembrolizumab (anti-PD1) in young patients with recurrent, progressive, or refractory brain tumors including ependymoma (NCT02359565) [126]. Additional novel checkpoint inhibitors such as the humanized IgG4 anti-PD-1 monoclonal antibody tiselizumab (BGB-A317) are under investigation (NCT02407990), with promising preliminary efficacy in stabilizing a case of extensive ependymoma with spinal and lung metastases for a duration of 18 months [127].

6.2.5 Macrophage modulation

Magrolimab is a first-in-class humanized IgG4 monoclonal antibody that blocks the macrophage checkpoint CD47, thereby inhibiting exhaustion of phagocytic macrophages. In a first-in-human basket trial of solid tumors (n = 84), magrolimab (Hu5F9-G4) was well tolerated [128]. No maximum tolerated dose was reached, and toxicities were mild to moderate, including transient anemia (57%), fatigue (64%), headache (50%), fever (45%), or chills (45%). An ongoing phase 1 trial of magrolimab in recurrent or progressive brain tumors is currently enrolling (NCT05169944) [129].

6.3 Future directions

Although extensive preclinical and clinical investigations have explored immunotherapy strategies in ependymoma, none are exclusively in the setting of NF2 mutations. Further investigation into the differences between sporadic and NF2-mediated ependymomas are necessary.

7. Conclusions

Immunotherapy has established itself as the fourth pillar of cancer therapy, following surgery, radiation, and chemotherapy. Thus far, there has been limited exploration into the potential of immunotherapy for NF2-associated tumors. No immunotherapy clinical trials have been conducted in vestibular schwannomas, a few studies are ongoing in meningiomas, and increasing clinical investigation is underway in ependymomas, borrowed predominantly from prior studies in glioblastoma. Potential strategies to harness the immune system include cancer vaccines, oncolytic viruses, dendritic cell vaccines, macrophage modulators, NK cell therapies, adoptive transfer, CAR T cells, checkpoint inhibitors and bispecific T cell engagers. Although current trials are not specifically restricted to patients with underlying NF2, future investigations may offer more insight in this unique population. Additional challenges include effective delivery of immunotherapy to the nervous system, reliable assessment of response versus progression through imaging and biomarkers, and rapid clinical trial accrual in this small and rare population. We hope that insights and limitations from our past experiences [130] will inform and pave the way for future advances toward a more effective treatment for NF2 associated tumors.

Acknowledgements

This work was supported by grant KL2TR001854 from the National Center for Advancing Translational Science (NCATS) of the U.S. National Institutes of Health. The content is solely the responsibility of the authors and does not necessarily represent the official views of the National Institutes of Health.

Conflict of interest

The authors declare no conflict of interest.

Author details

Shyam Patel[1], Thomas C. Chen[2] and Frances E. Chow[1*]

1 Departments of Neurological Surgery and Neurology, University of Southern California, Los Angeles, CA, USA

2 Department of Neurological Surgery, University of Southern California, Los Angeles, CA, USA

*Address all correspondence to: frances.chow@med.usc.edu

IntechOpen

© 2023 The Author(s). Licensee IntechOpen. This chapter is distributed under the terms of the Creative Commons Attribution License (http://creativecommons.org/licenses/by/3.0), which permits unrestricted use, distribution, and reproduction in any medium, provided the original work is properly cited. (cc) BY

References

[1] Neurofibromatosis. Conference statement. National Institutes of Health Consensus Development Conference. Archives of Neurology. 1988;**45**(5):575-578

[2] Evans DG, King AT, Bowers NL, Tobi S, Wallace AJ, Perry M, et al. Identifying the deficiencies of current diagnostic criteria for neurofibromatosis 2 using databases of 2777 individuals with molecular testing. Genetics in Medicine. 2019;**21**(7):1525-1533

[3] Plotkin SR, Messiaen L, Legius E, Pancza P, Avery RA, Blakeley JO, et al. Updated diagnostic criteria and nomenclature for neurofibromatosis type 2 and schwannomatosis: An international consensus recommendation. Genetics in Medicine. 2022;**24**(9):1967-1977

[4] Wilding A, Ingham SL, Lalloo F, Clancy T, Huson SM, Moran A, et al. Life expectancy in hereditary cancer predisposing diseases: An observational study. Journal of Medical Genetics. 2012;**49**(4):264-269

[5] Evans DG, Huson SM, Donnai D, Neary W, Blair V, Newton V, et al. A clinical study of type 2 neurofibromatosis. The Quarterly Journal of Medicine. 1992;**84**(304):603-618

[6] Baser ME, Evans DG, Jackler RK, Sujansky E, Rubenstein A. Neurofibromatosis 2, radiosurgery and malignant nervous system tumours. British Journal of Cancer. 2000;**82**(4):998

[7] Balasubramaniam A, Shannon P, Hodaie M, Laperriere N, Michaels H, Guha A. Glioblastoma multiforme after stereotactic radiotherapy for acoustic neuroma: Case report and review of the literature. Neuro-Oncology. 2007;**9**(4):447-453

[8] Rouleau GA, Wertelecki W, Haines JL, Hobbs WJ, Trofatter JA, Seizinger BR, et al. Genetic linkage of bilateral acoustic neurofibromatosis to a DNA marker on chromosome 22. Nature. 1987;**329**(6136):246-248

[9] Narod SA, Parry DM, Parboosingh J, Lenoir GM, Ruttledge M, Fischer G, et al. Neurofibromatosis type 2 appears to be a genetically homogeneous disease. American Journal of Human Genetics. 1992;**51**(3):486-496

[10] Phadnis S, Hagiwara M, Yaffe A, Mitchell C, Nicolaides T, Akshintala S, et al. Phase II study of axitinib in patients with neurofibromatosis type 2 and progressive vestibular schwannomas. Neuro-Oncology. 2020;**22**(Suppl 3):iii419

[11] Karajannis MA, Legault G, Hagiwara M, Ballas MS, Brown K, Nusbaum AO, et al. Phase II trial of lapatinib in adult and pediatric patients with neurofibromatosis type 2 and progressive vestibular schwannomas. Neuro-Oncology. 2012;**14**(9):1163-1170

[12] Goutagny S, Raymond E, Esposito-Farese M, Trunet S, Mawrin C, Bernardeschi D, et al. Phase II study of mTORC1 inhibition by everolimus in neurofibromatosis type 2 patients with growing vestibular schwannomas. Journal of Neuro-Oncology. 2015;**122**(2): 313-320

[13] ClinicalTrials.gov. A Study of Nilotinib in Growing Vestibular Schwannomas [Internet]. 2023. Available from: https://clinicaltrials.gov/ct2/show/NCT01201538 [Accessed: February 20, 2023].

[14] Welling DB, Collier KA, Burns SS, Oblinger JL, Shu E, Miles-Markley BA, et al. Early phase clinical studies of AR-42, a histone deacetylase inhibitor, for neurofibromatosis type 2-associated vestibular schwannomas and meningiomas. Laryngoscope Investigative Otolaryngology. 2021;**6**(5):1008-1019

[15] Collier KA, Valencia H, Newton H, Made EM, Sborov DW, Cavliere R, et al. A phase 1 trial of the histone deacetylase inhibitor AR-42 in patients with neurofibromatosis type 2-associated tumors and advanced solid malignancies. Cancer Chemotherapy and Pharmacology. 2021;**87**(5):599-611

[16] Plotkin SR, Halpin C, McKenna MJ, Loeffler JS, Batchelor TT, Barker FG 2nd. Erlotinib for progressive vestibular schwannoma in neurofibromatosis 2 patients. Otology & Neurotology. 2010;**31**(7):1135-1143

[17] Zhao Y, Liu P, Zhang N, Chen J, Landegger LD, Wu L, et al. Targeting the cMET pathway augments radiation response without adverse effect on hearing in NF2 schwannoma models. Proceedings of the National Academy of Sciences of the United States of America. 2018;**9**:E2077-E2084

[18] PlotkinS,AllenJ,Babovic-VuksanovicD, Dinh C, Nghiemphu L, Trippa L, et al. INTUITT-NF2, an adaptive platform-basket trial for neurofibromatosis 2 patients with progressive tumors: Interim results of the brigatinib treatment arm. Neuro-Oncology. 2022;**24**(s7):vii88

[19] Plotkin S, Jordan J, Beauchamp R, Muzikansky A, Stemmer-Rachamimov A, Ramesh V. A single arm phase 2 study of the dual mTORC1/mTORC2 inhibitor vistusertib provided on an intermittent schedule for neurofibromatosis 2 patients with progressive or symptomatic meningiomas. Neuro-Oncology. 2018;**20**(Suppl 6):vi19

[20] ClinicalTrials.gov. Trial of Selumetinib in Patients With Neurofibromatosis Type II Related Tumors (SEL-TH-1601) [Internet]. 2023. Available from: https://clinicaltrials.gov/ct2/show/NCT03095248 [Accessed: February 20, 2023]

[21] The Cancer Research Institute. FDA Approval Timeline [Internet]. 2023. Available from: https://www.cancerresearch.org/fda-approval-timeline-of-active-immunotherapies [Accessed: February 20, 2023]

[22] Sampson JH, Heimberger AB, Archer GE, Aldape KD, Friedman AH, Friedman HS, et al. Immunologic escape after prolonged progression-free survival with epidermal growth factor receptor variant III peptide vaccination in patients with newly diagnosed glioblastoma. Journal of Clinical Oncology. 2010;**28**(31):4722-4729

[23] Sampson JH, Aldape KD, Archer GE, Coan A, Desjardins A, Friedman AH, et al. Greater chemotherapy-induced lymphopenia enhances tumor-specific immune responses that eliminate EGFRvIII-expressing tumor cells in patients with glioblastoma. Neuro-Oncology. 2011;**13**(3):324-333

[24] Lai RK, Recht LD, Reardon DA, Paleologos N, Groves M, Rosenfeld MR, et al. Long-term follow-up of ACT III: A phase II trial of rindopepimut (CDX-110) in newly diagnosed glioblastoma. Neuro-Oncology. 2011;**13**(Suppl 3):iii34-iii40

[25] Reardon DA, Desjardins A, Vredenburgh JJ, O'Rourke DM, Tran DD, Fink KL, et al. Rindopepimut with bevacizumab for patients with relapsed

EGFRvIII-expressing glioblastoma (ReACT): Results of a double-blind randomized phase II trial. Clinical Cancer Research. 2020;**26**(7):1586-1594

[26] Weller M, Butowski N, Tran DD, Recht LD, Lim M, Hirte H, et al. Rindopepimut with temozolomide for patients with newly diagnosed, EGFRvIII-expressing glioblastoma (ACT IV): A randomised, double-blind, international phase 3 trial. The Lancet Oncology. 2017;**18**(10):1373-1385

[27] Desjardins A, Gromeier M, Herndon JE 2nd, Beaubier N, Bolognesi DP, Friedman AH, et al. Recurrent glioblastoma treated with recombinant poliovirus. The New England Journal of Medicine. 2018;**379**(2):150-161

[28] Rius-Rocabert S, García-Romero N, García A, Ayuso-Sacido A, Nistal-Villan E. Oncolytic virotherapy in glioma tumors. International Journal of Molecular Sciences. 2020;**21**(20):7604

[29] Liau LM, Ashkan K, Brem S, Campian JL, Trusheim JE, Iwamoto FM, et al. Association of autologous tumor lysate-loaded dendritic cell vaccination with extension of survival among patients with newly diagnosed and recurrent glioblastoma: A phase 3 prospective externally controlled cohort trial. JAMA Oncology. 2023;**9**(1):112-121

[30] Lewis D, Roncaroli F, Agushi E, Mosses D, Williams R, Li KL, et al. Inflammation and vascular permeability correlate with growth in sporadic vestibular schwannoma. Neuro-Oncology. 2019;**21**(3):314-325

[31] Liu J, Geng X, Hou J, Wu G. New insights into M1/M2 macrophages: Key modulators in cancer progression. Cancer Cell International. 2021;**21**(1):389

[32] Freud AG, Mundy-Bosse BL, Yu J, Caligiuri MA. The broad spectrum of human natural killer cell diversity. Immunity. 2017;**47**(5):820-833

[33] Siegler EL, Wang P. Preclinical models in chimeric antigen receptor-engineered T-cell therapy. Human Gene Therapy. 2018;**29**(5):534-546

[34] Brown CE, Alizadeh D, Starr R, Weng L, Wagner JR, Naranjo A, et al. Regression of glioblastoma after chimeric antigen receptor T-cell therapy. The New England Journal of Medicine. 2016;**375**(26):2561-2569

[35] Cloughesy TF, Mochizuki AY, Orpilla JR, Hugo W, Lee AH, Davidson TB, et al. Neoadjuvant anti-PD-1 immunotherapy promotes a survival benefit with intratumoral and systemic immune responses in recurrent glioblastoma. Nature Medicine. 2019;**25**(3):477-486

[36] Chow F, Mochizuki A, Lee A, Galvez M, Orpilla J, Everson R, et al. Validation of response to neoadjuvant anti-PD-1 immunotherapy in recurrent glioblastoma. Neuro-Oncology. 2020;**21**(6):vi4-vi5

[37] Kim JE, Patel MA, Mangraviti A, Kim ES, Theodros D, Velarde E, et al. Combination therapy with anti-PD-1, anti-TIM-3, and focal radiation results in regression of murine gliomas. Clinical Cancer Research. 2017;**23**(1):124-136

[38] Medawar PB. Immunity to homologous grafted skin; the fate of skin homografts transplanted to the brain, to subcutaneous tissue, and to the anterior chamber of the eye. British Journal of Experimental Pathology. 1948;**29**(1):58-69

[39] Iliff JJ, Wang M, Liao Y, Plogg BA, Peng W, Gundersen GA, et al. A

paravascular pathway facilitates CSF flow through the brain parenchyma and the clearance of interstitial solutes, including amyloid β. Science Translational Medicine. 2012;**4**(147):147ra111

[40] Louveau A, Smirnov I, Keyes TJ, Eccles JD, Rouhani SJ, Peske JD, et al. Structural and functional features of central nervous system lymphatic vessels. Nature. 2015;**523**(7560):337-341

[41] Iliff JJ, Nedergaard M. Is there a cerebral lymphatic system? Stroke. 2013;**44**(6 Suppl 1):S93-S95

[42] Cserr HF, Cooper DN, Suri PK, Patlak CS. Efflux of radiolabeled polyethylene glycols and albumin from rat brain. The American Journal of Physiology. 1981;**240**(4):F319-F328

[43] Johnston M, Zakharov A, Papaiconomou C, Salmasi G, Armstrong D. Evidence of connections between cerebrospinal fluid and nasal lymphatic vessels in humans, non-human primates and other mammalian species. Cerebrospinal Fluid Research. 2004;**1**(1):2

[44] Murtha LA, Yang Q, Parsons MW, Levi CR, Beard DJ, Spratt NJ, et al. Cerebrospinal fluid is drained primarily via the spinal canal and olfactory route in young and aged spontaneously hypertensive rats. Fluids and Barriers of the CNS. 2014;**11**:12

[45] Szentistvanyi I, Patlak CS, Ellis RA, Cserr HF. Drainage of interstitial fluid from different regions of rat brain. The American Journal of Physiology. 1984;**246**:F835-F844

[46] Weller RO, Djuanda E, Yow HY, Carare RO. Lymphatic drainage of the brain and the pathophysiology of neurological disease. Acta Neuropathologica. 2009;**117**:1-14

[47] Pardridge WM. CNS drug design based on principles of blood–brain barrier transport. Journal of Neurochemistry. 1998;**70**:1781-1792

[48] Pardridge WM. Blood–brain barrier delivery. Drug Discovery Today. 2007;**12**:54-61

[49] Coulie PG, Van den Eynde BJ, van der Bruggen P, Boon T. Tumour antigens recognized by T lymphocytes: At the core of cancer immunotherapy. Nature Reviews. Cancer. 2014;**14**(2):135-146

[50] Meléndez B, Van Campenhout C, Rorive S, Remmelink M, Salmon I, D'Haene N. Methods of measurement for tumor mutational burden in tumor tissue. Translational Lung Cancer Research. 2018;7(6):661-667

[51] McGranahan N, Furness AJS, Rosenthal R, Ramskov S, Lyngaa R, Kumar Saini S, et al. Clonal neoantigens elicit T cell immunoreactivity and sensitivity to immune checkpoint blockade. Science. 2016;**351**:1463-1469

[52] Alexandrov LB, Nik-Zainal S, Wedge DC, Aparicio SAJR, Behjati S, Biankin AV, et al. Signatures of mutational processes in human cancer. Nature. 2013;**500**:415-421

[53] Yarchoan M, Hopkins A, Jaffee EM. Tumor mutational burden and response rate to PD-1 inhibition. The New England Journal of Medicine. 2017;**377**:2500-2501

[54] Fusco M, Macaulay RJ, Forsyth PAJ, Walko CM. Detection of targetable somatic alterations in glioblastoma (GBM) and clinical impact. Journal of Clinical Oncology. *2019*;**37**:2058

[55] Li B et al. Comprehensive analyses of tumor immunity: Implications for cancer immunotherapy. Genome Biology. 2016;**17**:174

[56] Lee AH, Sun L, Mochizuki AY, Reynoso JG, Orpilla J, Chow F, et al. Neoadjuvant PD-1 blockade induces T cell and cDC1 activation but fails to overcome the immunosuppressive tumor associated macrophages in recurrent glioblastoma. Nature Communications. 2021;**12**(1):6938

[57] Lu Y, Ng AHC, Chow F, Everson RG, Helmink BA, Tetzlaff MT, et al. Resolution of tissue signatures of therapy response in patients with recurrent GBM treated with neoadjuvant anti-PD1. Nature Communications. 2021;**12**(1):4031

[58] Mochizuki A, Lee A, Orpilla J, Kienzler J, Galvez M, Chow F, et al. Myeloid populations and the effect of neoadjuvant PD-1 inhibition in the glioblastoma microenvironment: A surfaceomic and transcriptomic dissection at the single-cell level. Neuro-Oncology. 2019;**21**(Suppl 6):vi248

[59] Antoni NRE. Über Rückenmarkstumoren und Neurofibrome. Munich: JF Bergmann; 1920

[60] Rasmussen N, Bendtzen K, Thomsen J, Tos M. Specific cellular immunity in acoustic neuroma patients. Otolaryngology and Head and Neck Surgery. 1983;**91**(05):532-536

[61] Harker LA, Nysather J, Katz A. Immunologic detection of acoustic neuroma: Preliminary report. The Laryngoscope. 1978;**88**(5):802-807

[62] Rossi ML, Jones NR, Esiri MM, Havas L, Nakamura N, Coakham HB. Mononuclear cell infiltrate, HLA-Dr expression and proliferation in 37 acoustic schwannomas. Histology and Histopathology. 1990;**5**(4):427-432

[63] Archibald DJ, Neff BA, Voss SG, Splinter PL, Driscoll CL, Link MJ, et al. B7-H1 expression in vestibular schwannomas. Otology & Neurotology. 2010;**31**(6):991-997

[64] Dilwali S, Briët MC, Kao SY, Fujita T, Landegger LD, Platt MP, et al. Preclinical validation of anti-nuclear factor-kappa B therapy to inhibit human vestibular schwannoma growth. Molecular Oncology. 2015;**9**(7):1359-1370

[65] Taurone S, Bianchi E, Attanasio G, Di Gioia C, Ierinó R, Carubbi C, et al. Immunohistochemical profile of cytokines and growth factors expressed in vestibular schwannoma and in normal vestibular nerve tissue. Molecular Medicine Reports. 2015;**12**(1):737-745

[66] Constantin G, Piccio L, Bussini S, Pizzuti A, Scarpini E, Baron P, et al. Induction of adhesion molecules on human schwann cells by proinflammatory cytokines, an immunofluorescence study. Journal of the Neurological Sciences. 1999;**170**(2):124-130

[67] Breun M, Schwerdtfeger A, Martellotta DD. CXCR4: A new player in vestibular schwannoma pathogenesis. Oncotarget. 2018;**9**(11):9940-9950

[68] de Vries WM, Briaire-de Bruijn IH, van Benthem PPG, van der Mey AGL, Hogendoorn PCW. M-CSF and IL-34 expression as indicators for growth in sporadic vestibular schwannoma. Virchows Archiv. 2019;**474**(3):375-381

[69] Labit-Bouvier C, Crebassa B, Bouvier C, Andrac-Meyer L, Magnan J, Charpin C. Clinicopathologic growth factors in vestibular schwannomas: A morphological and immunohistochemical study of 69 tumours. Acta Oto-Laryngologica. 2000;**120**(08):950-954

[70] Schulz A, Büttner R, Hagel C, Baader SL, Kluwe L, Salamon J, et al. The

importance of nerve microenvironment for schwannoma development. Acta Neuropathologica. 2016;**132**(2):289-307

[71] de Vries M, Hogendoorn PCW, De Bruyn IB, Malessy MJA, Van Der Mey AGL. Intratumoral hemorrhage, vessel density, and the inflammatory reaction contribute to volume increase of sporadic vestibular schwannomas. Virchows Archiv. 2012;**460**(6):629-636

[72] de Vries M, Briaire-de Bruijn I, Malessy MJ, de Bruïne SF, van der Mey AG, Hogendoorn PC. Tumor-associated macrophages are related to volumetric growth of vestibular schwannomas. Otology & Neurotology. 2013;**34**(2):347-352

[73] Tamura R, Morimoto Y, Sato M. Difference in the hypoxic immunosuppressive microenvironment of patients with neurofibromatosis type 2 schwannomas and sporadic schwannomas. Journal of Neuro-Oncology. 2020;**146**(02):265-273

[74] Hannan CJ, Lewis D, O'Leary C, Donofrio CA, Evans DG, Roncaroli F, et al. The inflammatory microenvironment in vestibular schwannoma. Neuro-Oncology Advances. 2020;**2**:vdaa023

[75] Tamura R, Morimoto Y, Sato M, Kuranari Y, Oishi Y, Kosugi K, et al. Difference in the hypoxic immunosuppressive microenvironment of patients with neurofibromatosis type 2 schwannomas and sporadic schwannomas. Neuro-Oncology. 2020;**146**:265-273

[76] Nisenbaum E, Misztalm C, Szczupak M, Thielhelm T, Peña S, Mei C, et al. Tumor-associated macrophages in vestibular schwannoma and relationship to hearing. OTO Open. 2021;**5**:2473974X211059111

[77] Tamura R, Tanaka T, Akasaki Y, Murayama Y, Yoshida K, Sasaki H. The role of vascular endothelial growth factor in the hypoxic and immunosuppressive tumor microenvironment: Perspectives for therapeutic implications. Medical Oncology. 2019;**37**:2

[78] Tamura R, Fujioka M, Morimoto Y, Ohara K, Kosugi K, Oishi Y, et al. A VEGF receptor vaccine demonstrates preliminary efficacy in neurofibromatosis type 2. Nature Communications. 2019;**10**:5758

[79] Jacobs JF, Idema AJ, Bol KF, Nierkens S, Grauer OM, Wesseling P, et al. Regulatory T cells and the PD-L1/PD-1 pathway mediate immune suppression in malignant human brain tumors. Neuro-Oncology. 2009;**11**:394-402

[80] Li Z, Liu X, Guo R, Wang P. TIM-3 plays a more important role than PD-1 in the functional impairments of cytotoxic T cells of malignant schwannomas. Tumor Biology. 2017;**39**:1010428317698352

[81] Perry A, Graffeo CS, Carlstrom LP, Raghunathan A, Driscoll CLW, Neff BA, et al. Predominance of M1 subtype among tumor-associated macrophages in phenotypically aggressive sporadic vestibular schwannoma. Neurosurgery. 2020;**133**(6):1637-1645

[82] Wang S, Liechty B, Patel S, Weber JS, Hollmann TJ, Snuderl M, et al. Programmed death ligand 1 expression and tumor infiltrating lymphocytes in neurofibromatosis type 1 and 2 associated tumors. Neuro-Oncology. 2018;**138**(1):183-190

[83] Chang JH, Tseng CY, Lee JH, Hsueh C. Anti-PD-1 immune checkpoint inhibition for vestibular schwannoma therapy. OncoImmunology. 2018;**7**(12):e1469564

[84] Guo Y, Chen Y, Liu X, Min JJ, Tan W, Zheng JH. Targeted cancer immunotherapy with genetically engineered oncolytic *Salmonella typhimurium*. Cancer Letters. 2020;**469**:102-110

[85] Zheng JH, Nguyen VH, Jiang SN, Park SH, Tan W, Hong SH, et al. Two-step enhanced cancer immunotherapy with engineered Salmonella typhimurium secreting heterologous flagellin. Science Translational Medicine. 2017;**9**(376):eaak9537

[86] Yang M, Xu J, Wang Q, Zhang AQ, Wang K. An obligatory anaerobic Salmonella typhimurium strain redirects M2 macrophages to the M1 phenotype. Oncology Letters. 2018;**15**(3):3918-3922

[87] Ahmed SG, Oliva G, Shao M, Wang X, Mekalanos JJ, Brenner GJ. Intratumoral injection of schwannoma with attenuated Salmonella typhimurium induces antitumor immunity and controls tumor growth. Proceedings of the National Academy of Sciences of the United States of America. 2022;**119**(24):e2202719119

[88] Proctor DT, Huang J, Lama S, Albakr A, Van Marle G, Sutherland GR. Tumor-associatedmacrophageinfiltration in meningioma. Neuro-Oncology Advances. 2019;**1**(01):1-10

[89] Rossi ML, Cruz Sanchez F, Hughes JT, Esiri MM, Coakham HB. Immunocytochemical study of the cellular immune response in meningiomas. Journal of Clinical Pathology. 1988;**41**:314-319

[90] Bo L, Mork SJ, Nyland H. An immunohistochemical study of mononuclear cells in meningiomas. Neuropathology and Applied Neurobiology. 1992;**18**:548-558

[91] Asai J, Suzuki R, Fujimoto T, Suzuki T, Nakagawa N, Nagashima G, et al. Fluorescence automatic cell sorter and immunohistochemical investigation of CD68-positive cells in meningioma. Clinical Neurology and Neurosurgery. 1999;**101**:229-234

[92] Pinton L, Solito S, Masetto E, Vettore M, Cane S, Puppa AD, et al. Immunosuppressive activity of tumor-infiltrating myeloid cells in patients with meningioma. Oncoimmunology. 2018;**7**:e1440931

[93] Domingues PH, Teodósio C, Ortiz J. Immunophenotypic identification and characterization of tumor cells and infiltrating cell populations in meningiomas. The American Journal of Pathology. 2012;**181**(05):1749-1761

[94] Stein M, Keshav S, Harris N, Gordon S. Interleukin 4 potently enhances murine macrophage mannose receptor activity: A marker of alternative immunologic macrophage activation. The Journal of Experimental Medicine. 1992;**176**(01):287-292

[95] Fang L, Lowther DE, Meizlish ML, Anderson RC, Bruce JN, Devine L, et al. The immune cell infiltrate populating meningiomas is composed of mature, antigen-experienced T and B cells. Neuro-Oncology. 2013;**15**:1479-1490

[96] Du Z, Abedalthagafi M, Aizer AA, Mchenry AR, Sun HH, Bray MA, et al. Increased expression of the immune modulatory molecule PD-L1 (CD274) in anaplastic meningioma. Oncotarget. 2015;**6**:4704-4716

[97] Proctor DT, Patel Z, Lama S, Resch L, Van Marle G, Sutherland GR. Identification of PD-L2, B7-H3 and CTLA-4 immune checkpoint proteins in genetic subtypes of meningioma. Oncoimmunology. 2019;**8**:e1512943

[98] Baia GS, Caballero OL, Ho JS, Zhao Q, Cohen T, Binder ZA, et al. NY-ESO-1 expression in meningioma suggests a rationale for new immunotherapeutic approaches. Cancer Immunology Research. 2013;**1**:296-302

[99] Han SJ, Reis G, Kohanbash G, Shrivastav S, Magill ST, Molinaro AM, et al. Expression and prognostic impact of immune modulatory molecule PD-L1 in meningioma. Neuro-Oncology. 2016;**130**:543-552

[100] Deng J, Ma M, Wang D, Zhu H, Hua L, Sun S, et al. Expression and clinical significance of immune checkpoint regulator B7-H3 (CD276) in human meningioma. World Neurosurgery. 2019;**135**:e12-e18

[101] Kaba SE, DeMonte F, Bruner JM, Kyritsis AP, Jaeckle KA, Levin V, et al. The treatment of recurrent unresectable and malignant meningiomas with interferon alpha-2B. Neurosurgery. 1997;**40**:271-275

[102] Chamberlain MC, Glantz MJ. Interferon-alpha for recurrent World Health Organization grade 1 intracranial meningiomas. Cancer. 2008;**113**:2146-2151

[103] Chamberlain MC. IFN-a for recurrent surgery- and radiation-refractory high-grade meningioma: A retrospective case series. CNS Oncology. 2013;**2**:227-235

[104] Brastianos PK, Kim AE, Giobbie-Hurder A, Lee EQ, Wang N, Eichler AF, et al. Phase 2 study of pembrolizumab in patients with recurrent and residual high-grade meningiomas. Nature Communications. 2022;**13**(1):1325

[105] Bi WL, Nayak L, Meredith DM, Driver J, Du Z, Hoffman S, et al. Activity of PD-1 blockade with nivolumab among patients with recurrent atypical/anaplastic meningioma: Phase II trial results. Neuro-Oncology. 2022;**24**(1):101-113

[106] ClinicalTrials.gov. T Cell Receptor Immunotherapy Targeting NY-ESO-1 for Patients With NY-ESO-1 Expressing Cancer [Internet]. 2023. Available from: https://clinicaltrials.gov/ct2/show/study/NCT01967823 [Accessed: February 20, 2023]

[107] Sun M, Orpilla J, Contreras E, Treger J, Molaie D, Tsang J, et al. Systemic adoptive transfer immunotherapy with TCR-transduced T-cells targeting NY-ESO-1 for meningioma. Neuro-Oncology. 2019;**21**(Suppl 6):vi129-vi130

[108] Nam SJ, Kim YH, Park JE, Ra YS, Khang SK, Cho YH, et al. Tumor-infiltrating immune cell subpopulations and programmed death ligand 1 (PD-L1) expression associated with clinicopathological and prognostic parameters in ependymoma. Cancer Immunology, Immunotherapy. 2019;**68**(2):305-318

[109] Yeung JT, Hamilton RL, Okada H, Jakacki RI, Pollack IF. Increased expression of tumor-associated antigens in pediatric and adult ependymomas: Implication for vaccine therapy. Neuro-Oncology. 2013;**111**(2):103-111

[110] Hatano M, Eguchi J, Tatsumi T, Kuwashima N, Dusak JE, Kinch MS, et al. EphA2 as a glioma-associated antigen: A novel target for glioma vaccines. Neoplasia. 2005;**7**(8):717-722

[111] Morris KA, Afridi SK, Evans G, Hensiek AE, McCabe MG, Kellett M, et al. The response of spinal cord ependymomas to bevacizumab in patients with neurofibromatosis

type 2. Journal of Neurosurgery. Spine. 2017;**26**(4):474-482

[112] Farschtschi S, Merker VL, Wolf D, Schuhmann M, Blakeley J, Plotkin SR, et al. Bevacizumab treatment for symptomatic spinal ependymomas in neurofibromatosis type 2. Acta Neurologica Scandinavica. 2016;**133**(6):475-480

[113] Donson AM, Birks DK, Barton VN, Wei Q, Kleinschmidt-Demasters BK, Handler MH, et al. Immune gene and cell enrichment is associated with a good prognosis in ependymoma. Journal of Immunology. 2009;**183**(11):7428-7440

[114] ClinicalTrials.gov. A Pilot Study of SurVaxM in Children Progressive or Relapsed Medulloblastoma, High Grade Glioma, Ependymoma and Newly Diagnosed Diffuse Intrinsic Pontine Glioma [Internet]. 2023. Available from: https://clinicaltrials.gov/ct2/show/NCT04978727 [Accessed: February 20, 2023]

[115] Preusser M, Wolfsberger S, Czech T, Slavc I, Budka H, Hainfellner JA. Survivin expression in intracranial ependymomas and its correlation with tumor cell proliferation and patient outcome. American Journal of Clinical Pathology. 2005;**124**(4):543-549

[116] Ahluwalia MS, Reardon DA, Abad AP, Curry WT, Wong ET, Figel SA, et al. Phase IIa study of SurVaxM plus adjuvant temozolomide for newly diagnosed glioblastoma. Journal of Clinical Oncology. 2023;**41**(7):1453-1465

[117] ClinicalTrials.gov. Immunotherapy for Recurrent Ependymomas in Children Using Tumor Antigen Peptides With Imiquimod [Internet]. 2023. Available from: https://clinicaltrials.gov/ct2/show/NCT01795313 [Accessed: February 20, 2023]

[118] ClinicalTrials.gov. HSV G207 in Children With Recurrent or Refractory Cerebellar Brain Tumors [Internet]. 2023. Available from: https://clinicaltrials.gov/ct2/show/NCT03911388 [Accessed: February 20, 2023]

[119] Totsch SK, Schlappi C, Kang KD, Ishizuka AS, Lynn GM, Fox B, et al. Oncolytic herpes simplex virus immunotherapy for brain tumors: Current pitfalls and emerging strategies to overcome therapeutic resistance. Oncogene. 2019;**38**(34):6159-6171

[120] Nellan A, Griesinger A, Witt D, Donson A, Amani V, Foreman NK. Study of anti-HER2 CAR T cells in the immunosuppressive ependymoma tumor microenvironment. Neuro-Oncology. 2018;**20**(Suppl 2):i80

[121] ClinicalTrials.gov. HER2-specific Chimeric Antigen Receptor (CAR) T Cells for Children With Ependymoma [Internet]. 2023. Available from: https://clinicaltrials.gov/ct2/show/NCT04903080 [Accessed: February 20, 2023]

[122] ClinicalTrials.gov. Brain Tumor-Specific Immune Cells (IL13Ralpha2-CAR T Cells) for the Treatment of Leptomeningeal Glioblastoma, Ependymoma, or Medulloblastoma [Internet]. 2023. Available from: https://clinicaltrials.gov/ct2/show/NCT04903080 [Accessed: February 20, 2023]

[123] Kawakami M, Kawakami K, Takahashi S, Abe M, Puri RK. Analysis of interleukin-13 receptor alpha2 expression in human pediatric brain tumors. Cancer. 2004;**101**(5):1036-1042

[124] Nellan A, Donson A, Calhoun J, Griesinger A, Fry T, Foreman N. Evaluation of CAR T cells in epenydmoma. Neuro-Oncology. 2020;**22**(Suppl 3):iii364

[125] Hegde M, Mukherjee M, Grada Z, Pignata A, Landi D, Navai SA, et al. Tandem CAR T cells targeting HER2 and IL13Rα2 mitigate tumor antigen escape. The Journal of Clinical Investigation. 2016;**126**(8):3036-3052

[126] ClinicalTrials.gov. Pembrolizumab in Treating Younger Patients With Recurrent, Progressive, or Refractory High-Grade Gliomas, Diffuse Intrinsic Pontine Gliomas, Hypermutated Brain Tumors, Ependymoma or Medulloblastoma [Internet]. 2023. Available from: https://clinicaltrials.gov/ct2/show/NCT02359565 [Accessed: February 20, 2023]

[127] Tapia Rico G, Townsend A, Price T, Patterson K. Metastatic myxopapillary ependymoma treated with immunotherapy achieving durable response. BML Case Reports. 2020;**13**(12):e236242

[128] Sikic BI, Lakhani N, Patnaik A, Shah SA, Chandana SR, Rasco D, et al. First-in-human, first-in-class phase I trial of the anti-CD47 antibody Hu5F9-G4 in patients with advanced cancers. Journal of Clinical Oncology. 2019;**37**(12):946-953

[129] ClinicalTrials.gov. Magrolimab in Children and Adults with Recurrent or Progressive Malignant Brain Tumors (PNOC025) [Internet]. 2023. Available from: https://clinicaltrials.gov/ct2/show/NCT05169944 [Accessed: February 20, 2023]

[130] Chuntova P, Chow F, Galvez M, Watchmaker P, Prins R, Okada H, et al. Unique challenges for glioblastoma immunotherapy: Discussions across neuro-oncology and non-neuro-oncology experts in cancer immunology. Neuro-Oncology. 2021;**23**(3):356-375

Chapter 4

Therapeutic Approach to Plexiform Neurofibromas

Elisabetta Basso, Enrico Opocher, Franco Bassetto, Martina Grigatti, Alvise Montanari, Stefano Ferraresi and Federica Chiara

Abstract

Neurofibromatosis (NF1) is a rare genetic disease that predisposes to tumors in the peripheral and central nervous systems and other neoplasms. Neurofibromas are complex benign tumors involving various cell types. Among them, plexiform neurofibromas are locally invasive peripheral nerve sheath tumors (PNs) that can cause disfigurement and functional limitations. Based on histopathological and magnetic resonance imaging (MRI) data, PNs display variable morphology and behavior. The appearance of distinct nodular lesions (DNLs) in PNs raises concerns about an increased risk of transformation into malignant peripheral nerve sheath tumors (MPNSTs). Surgery represents the primary treatment option for NF1-related PN, although recently, specific targeted agents, that is, MEK inhibitors, have been shown to be partially effective. Several surgical techniques have been proposed for PNs to decrease intraoperative bleeding and facilitate tumor excision of either diffuse PNs or rapidly growing nodular PN. However, despite improving surgical methods, complete tumor excision can be achieved in only a few cases. In this frame, it emerges evident that searching for appropriate surgical and pharmacological treatments for neurofibromas is a priority challenge. In this chapter, we will review current treatments approved by the scientific/clinical community, emphasizing the most recent progress in this field.

Keywords: neurofibromatosis type 1, neurofibroma, treatment, neurofibroma surgery, tumour progression, MPNST, MEK inhibitors, Selumetinib

1. Introduction

Neurofibromatosis type 1 (NF1; OMIM 613113) is an autosomal dominant disease affecting approximately 1 in 2500 individuals worldwide. NF1 is associated with cutaneous, neurologic, and orthopedic symptoms, some of which are progressive and lead to significant morbidity or mortality. The latest consensus has been reached for diagnosis and resumed in the guidelines for neurofibromatosis type 1 recently published [1, 2]. Among the clinical features considered was the development of characteristic tumors such as neurofibromas or gliomas; the presence of cutaneous findings including cafè au lait macules (CALMs), skinfold freckling, juvenile

 IntechOpen

xanthogranulomas, and nevus anemicus, ophthalmologic markers such as Lisch nodules and choroidal abnormalities and the occurrence of characteristic osseous lesions such as sphenoid wing dysplasia, scoliosis, anterolateral bowing of the lower leg, pseudarthrosis.

This syndrome is caused by pathogenic variants in the NF1 gene encoding neurofibromin enzyme (Nf1). Nf1 operates as a GTPase-activating protein (GAP) that negatively regulates the RAS/MAPK pathway activity by accelerating the hydrolysis of RAS-bound GTP [3]. All alterations in the NF1 gene result in loss-of-function of the Nf1, causing an uncontrolled cell proliferation and growth. The neurofibromin haploinsufficiency, and the consequent Ras proto-oncogene hyperactivation, make NF1 a tumor predisposing disease [4]. Nf1 affected individuals, display increased risk of certain cancers, including female breast cancer <50 years, gastrointestinal, neuro-endocrine brain and hematopoietic tumors [5–7].

The most relevant manifestation of NF1 is the appearance of tumors in both the Central (CNS) and Peripheral Nervous Systems (PNS) as gliomas and neurofibromas, respectively. Of the tumors involving the nervous system, peripheral nerve sheath tumors (cutaneous and plexiform neurofibromas) are frequently found in between 30 and 60% of subjects with NF1, depending on diagnostic modalities (symptomatic Vs screening) and can present at a various age range from congenital to young adulthood (median age 5.5 years). In addition, 8–13% of individuals harboring a PN can develop a malignant peripheral nerve sheath tumor (MPNSTs) [8, 9]. The appearance of distinct nodular lesions (DNLs) in PNs raises clinical concerns, as these changes are correlated to increased risk of transformation into Atypical Neurofibroma (AN) or MPNSTs [10], the prognosis of which is ominous due to delayed diagnosis, early metastasis, and poor response to systemic therapy [11]. Atypical neurofibromatous neoplasms of uncertain biological potential (ANNUBPs), are potentially premalignant lesions with unique biology still under investigation but are often characterized by specific histological features including cytological atypia, hypercellularity, loss of neurofibroma architecture, and an increased mitotic index [12]. Also ANNUBP can be associated with additional somatic genetic events such as heterozygous or homozygous loss of CDKN2A/B in addition to NF1 alteration [13] and often display a more aggressive growth behavior. Furthermore, individuals with AN/ANNUBP are at higher risk for the development of malignant peripheral nerve sheath tumors (MPNSTs), with a 33% incidence in one study versus the cumulative MPNST risk of 15.8% in the general NF1 population [6, 14].

Even though a large number of histological changes between PNs and MPNSTs has been described, a clear molecular definition of the stepwise characteristics of PN evolution towards MPNSTs is currently under investigation [15, 16]. The effort to fully elucidate the development and progression of these tumors, finalized to identify genes suitable for diagnostic markers and pharmacological targets, is made even more difficult by their structural heterogeneity and a complex tumor-host interaction.

Neurofibromas arise within nerves and comprise multiple cell types, including Schwann cells, fibroblasts, perineural cells, mast cells, and macrophages [17]. The PNST development requires both biallelic loss of NF1 in Schwann cells, and a haplo-insufficient microenvironment. Whereas the knowledge on the molecular basis of Schwann cell transformation is increasing, a deeper understanding of the exact contribution of the microenvironment in the Schwann cells neoplastic transformation [18] it is still elusive. The current concept in the NF1 field states that the tumorigenic proliferation of Nf1 haplo-insufficient Schwann cells depends on an inflammatory milieu triggering a powerful burst of mixed mitogenic signals from both collagen-secreting fibroblasts and pericytes stimulated by mast cells [19]. A considerable amount of data speak in favor of this pro-inflammatory model, in primis the discovery that mast cell have a central role in sustaining chronic inflammation, cell proliferation, and potent extracellular matrix deposition (ECM) leading to fibrotic tissue deposition; however, this model does not entirely fulfill the molecular signature proper of "tumorigenic" cells able to grow in the absence of basal membrane binding, possessing higher proliferative potential and own metabolism [17] and further investigation are required to fully understand how microenvironmental cells contribute to Schwann cell transformation.

In general, PNs are characterized by a slow-growing behavior tending to exhaust after a definite period of time. In addition, many PN can manifest prolonged quiescent phases, or sometimes even undergo a spontaneous partial regression, rendering its natural history often unpredictable [20].

From a prospective NF1-PN study ("NCI natural history") [21] the median PN volume change was +21.3%/year. Other studies suggested that infants or young children at PN diagnosis tend to present with more rapidly growing lesions compared to young adults [11, 20, 22].

While PNs may be asymptomatic, a proportion of PNs can lead to various morbidities, ranging from disfigurement, pain, functional motor-sensitive deficits, which can also be associated with life-threatening complications such as bleeding and vital structures (e.g., airways) obstruction.

In most cases, stable PN not causing morbidity should be observed, as they may never progress or cause symptoms and an active intervention should be offered only to those patients who manifest progressive growth over time causing significant symptoms which cannot be treated otherwise (e.g. pain medications ineffective) [23].

Furthermore, as morbidity is often secondary to the PN anatomical distribution, some locations (e.g., paraspinal, orbital, neck) may cause more symptoms than others (limbs, pelvis) and more often require an active treatment, irrespectively from their actual size.

PNs rapidly growing (>20% increase in volume in the prior year) are painful and with high risk of malignant transformation, thus should be considered for treatment [23]. In addition, PNs can exert a mass effect, compressing nearby structures (such as the trachea or blood vessels), and either stimulate bone growth or lead to bone erosion. PNs can also cause spinal cord compression, weakness, cranial neuropathy, disfigurement, and pain.

Although surgical treatment is the only curative treatment option, and it is indicated for symptomatic PNs, the tumor's complete removal is frequently not possible or associated with severe morbidity, especially in deep-seated tumors involving multiple nerves [24]. For instance, diffuse PNs spread extensively along connective tissue and surrounding normal tissue structures with indistinct borders, whereas nodular lesions are well-demarcated. Also, PNs have a rich vascular network and can bleed profusely during surgery.

Several surgical techniques have been proposed for PNs to decrease intraoperative bleeding and facilitate tumor excision of either diffuse PNs or rapidly growing nodular PN (DNL) [25, 26]; however, despite the improvement in surgical methods, reports on post-surgical outcomes suggest that complete tumor excision can be achieved in only low rate of cases (about 10–15%). Sometimes PN re-growth occurs in those who underwent either partial or subtotal resection [27, 28].

In this chapter, we will provide an overview of the most recent advances of tumor biology knowledge and treatment of neurofibromatosis derived peripheral tumors.

1.1 Non-surgical management of NF1-associated plexiform neurofibroma (PNs)

About 85–95% of PN are considered inoperable. Most of the times a complete surgery is not feasible due to the PN intimate anatomy and growth within the nerve fascicles as well as a significant vascularity leading to an increased risk of bleeding. Moreover, PN regrowth is frequent after incomplete surgery, particularly in young children, therefore any benefit of debulking surgery should be carefully balanced against risks.

Consequently, non-surgical treatment has been historically used to treated inoperable and symptomatic PN.

Unfortunately, until recent times, multiple trials have so far failed to identify any active agent against inoperable and symptomatic PN representing thus a clearly unmet medical need for a significant proportion of NF1-PNs.

First Roberston in 2012 published a phase II trial with series of 23 children or adults with NF1-PN in which 6/23 (26%; 95% CI: 10–48%) experienced ≥20% decrease in volume of one or more plexiform tumors and 30% had symptomatic improvement. Main predictive factors for Imatinib response were a smaller tumor (<20 cm^3 volume), head and neck location, while age was not predictive of response [29].

Few years later Weiss et al, published their experience (n = 46) on a phase II trial with the mTOR inhibitor Sirolimus, which showed Median TTP was 15.4 months compared to the historical placebo cohort (tipifarnib trial) of 11.9 months. No subjects achieved a partial response, and the largest volume decrease was 17%. Overall, Sirulimus was well tolerated (stomatitis, increased liver and cholesterol level) and it appeared as a reasonable alternative to imatinib with the advantage of a liquid formulation available [30].

Another trial with peg-interferon-alfa-2b compared to placebo also showed minimal response rate [31].

A tremendous advance in understanding of NF1 PN pathophysiology was only possible with the use of pre-clinical mouse model of NF1 mimicking patients' tumors, particularly those from N. Ratner's group and NCI (Bethesda) and allowing to test biological-based pre-clinical drug screening. These advances have rapidly identified the MAPK pathway signaling as the main driver of NF1-PN, focusing on MEK as an actionable target of MAPK downstream pathway, which subsequently led to the pre-clinical testing of MEK inhibitors in mouse models showing a remarkable and unprecedented response rate with significant tumor shrinkage in PN models [32, 33].

Following such preclinical evidence provided, a phase I/II trial (SPRINT) was launched at NCI testing a selective orally available MEK1–2 inhibitor currently under development for other indications (uveal melanoma), named Selumetinib [22]. Volumetric MRI assessments and functional outcomes such as quality of life were included in the study methods as primary and secondary outcomes respectively.

The exceptional response rate for a phase I trial, with a volumetric Partial Response (PR) of 20% volume reduction in 71% of the 50 enrolled children which was confirmed by the phase II data (PR = 68%) with relatively favorable toxicity profile [34]. A reduction of PN volume by a median change of 27.9% (−55.1% – +2.2%) was documented in the SPRINT trial. Median time to initial response, cycles (range) was 8 monthly cycles (range 4–20), and time to best response, was 16 cycles (range 4–36) suggesting that many patients tended to respond many months or even years after Selumetinib initiation. Progression-free survival (PFS) at 3 years after therapy start was of 84%. Mean duration of treatment was 24 months. However, at the time of analysis 23/50 (46%) children remained on treatment for a median of 4 years, experiencing a durable and/or ongoing response.

From the cohort of 50 children with NF1-PN suffering from a median of 3 target morbidities at baseline, before treatment. A functional effect was also demonstrated, including a significant improvement/amelioration of patient's symptoms, including pain, disfigurement, and quality of life, as well as an objective improvement in strength, range of motion and pulmonary function based on REiNS standardized response criteria.

Based on the SPRINT data on safety, radiological and clinical efficacy, Selumetinib (Koselugo) at the doses of 25 mg/m^2 BID has been now granted approval from FDA and EMA as the first licensed drug in children aged 2 or more, with NF1 and inoperable and symptomatic PN. Despite at present Koselugo can be only offered to those children able to swallow capsules, a currently ongoing phase I/II trial is evaluating an alternative sprinkle formulation in young children (>1 year) and will likely extend its indication to younger children not able to swallow capsules.

An additional stratum from the SPRINT trial evaluated the role of preventive use of Selumetinib in children with NF1-PN at risk of developing severe symptoms and showed similar efficacy (PR = 72%) and absence of symptoms during treatment and rate of volumetric shrinkage (−32,7, range − 16,8 to − 39,7%). From this specific subgroup of asymptomatic PN, younger patients were more likely to respond in terms of radiological tumor shrinkage when compared to older children suggesting a potential extended indication to start Selumetinib early in selected young children at risk, and before they develop PN-related symptoms [34].

1.2 Selumetinib real world data and ongoing studies

After its approval in US, UK ad EU, few retrospective cases series based on Early Access Program and compassionate use have contributed with real world data, including large institutional series from Espirito Santo et al. [35] in which all but one among the 19 patients who were treated with Selumetinib had a sustained clinical and/or radiological response mainly within the first 2–3 months from start.

Also, Cacchione et al. [36] from 13 patients (7 males, 6 females) -median age 3 yr-treated with either selumetinib [12] or Tranetinib (1) documented a PR rate of 23%, with a median time to onset of response to treatment of 12 cycles (6–30 range). All other patients were stable (SD = 69%) except in one case who had a rapid progression, and who was subsequently diagnosed with a malignant nerve sheath tumor (MPNST). A smaller series from Baldo et al. showed PN reduction of >20% in 16 out of 17 PN (94%). One PN remained stable and no PN progressed while on active treatment. Mean follow-up was relatively short (12 months) at the time of publication [37].

In addition to the SPRINT study, other Selumetinib trials are currently ongoing in US, UK or Europe. In adults, KOMET randomized trial of Selumetinib against placebo is open and enrolling patients with symptomatic and inoperable PN (NCT04924608). Moreover, a PASS (post authorization safety)- study will evaluate long-term Koselugo safety and other possible side effects including endocrine function in children. Two trials are evaluating alternative dosing, either intermittent (5 days on/2 days off, UK-GOSH (NCT 03326388) or a lower dose maintenance phase (US only, MJ Fisher personal communication) both aiming at optimizing treatment compliance and long-term tolerability.

1.3 Other MEKi efficacy data

Other MEKi have been tested against NF1-PN in other ongoing or more recently completed trials (cancel). One of the most relevant is the phase II trial (TRAM-01) including 46 children treated with a median of 16 months of Trametinib, a capsules and liquid formulation available MEKi, and showing that 17 out of 28 evaluable children with NF1-PN had a confirmed PR (60%) and a median decrease of - 30% as documented from a semi-automated volumetric calculation. In the meanwhile, Ronsley et al. [38] published their experience with Trametinib compassionate use showing response in 3/6 pediatric patients with NF1-PN.

Caution in direct comparison of various MEKi studies as study design, outcome measure, and enrolment criteria were slightly different by age, progressive/non progressive prior to start. Therefore, given the lack of direct comparison between various MEKi used to treat PN, it is not possible to assign a clear superiority of any MEKi at current stage.

With this in mind, other agents have shown promising data against NF1-PN both in children, such as the MEK inhibitors Binimetinib (19 children 2–16 yr., and a PR rate of 74%) or Mirdametinib (19 young adults 16–25 yr. and PR 42%, SD 53%, PD 5%) or Cabozantinib, a multiTKI targeting c-Kit, VEGFR2, MET, RET, FLT3 which was associated with a PR of 42% in 19 adults (>16 yr) with NF1-PN [39–41].

1.4 Selumetinib and other MEKi toxicities

Side effects from selumetinib were overall mild, with 10% who interrupted treatment due to intolerable or recurrent toxicities, but up to 30% of patients required in a dose reduction.

Notably, there were no AEs resulting in patient death and side effects were always reversible with drug interruption. Most frequently encountered and clinically detectable adverse effects (AE) were predominantly skin toxicity such as follicular or acneiform rash, paronychia in 52–58% (grade I/II) and 4–10% (Gr 3) often presenting within the first 2weeks of initiation of therapy and gastrointestinal side effects such as nausea, abdominal pain, diarrhea and, less frequently vomiting. In addition, elevation of creatinine kinase was frequently seen during monitoring of blood tests, but most often asymptomatic and not requiring any active intervention or drug interruption [42].

The most serious dose-limiting side effects of MEK inhibitors may involve cardiac- with decrease of ejection fraction, which was reported in 6–10% of children from SPRINT trial. Differently from the adult series, ophthalmic- with retinal fluid and detachment-toxicity was not reported within the SPRINT dataset [32, 42, 43].

Main side effects from Trametinib were similar to other MEKi, and including skin, gastrointestinal toxicities and asymptomatic CPK elevation, generally mild and manageable with an adequate supportive care or dose interruption and further adjustments.

While various MEKi seem to share a class-effect of similar toxicities, potential differences in frequency and severity of side effects may perhaps be due to the specific dose needed to achieve response for each MEKi.

A preventive strategy as well as regular monitoring of AE are of paramount importance as AEs are frequent and might require dose adjustments and dose reductions, due to AEs or other reasons, can lead to PN regrowth. Prevention of side-effects since the very first start of MEKi, particularly in high-risk subjects such as post-pubertal and young adolescent patients is a key factor to potentially help maintaining a durable response [23].

Other relevant aspects of MEKi treatment: Optimal duration, events after interruption, prevention of malignant degeneration.

While in the SPRINT trial treatment with Selumetinib was planned for an undetermined period of duration, limited to 24 months in case of stable disease only, long-term data available from a subset of patients showed that 23/50 (46%) patients remained on treatment beyond the initial 24 months period of scheduled treatment phase (Median TTP: 36 cycles, range 16–48), thus adding useful information regarding effect durability and long-term safety and tolerability. ORR and safety profile were confirmed. Furthermore, it was shown that among those patients who interrupted treatment, a proportion of cases with PN regrowth was seen, after a median of 3–5 months from interruption [32].

In addition, from the Trametinib TRAM-01 trial out of the 36 patients (80%) who discontinued treatment after the planned 18 months initial duration, 7 (19,4%) suffered from PN progression after a median of 6.1 months (range 5.2–17,9) from end of Trametinib, the majority of whom were successfully rechallenged with Trametinib [44].

While these data do not provide a clear nor evidence-based indication on the optimal duration of treatment with various MEKi it appears clear that interrupting it too early may lead to PN symptomatic regrowth, particularly in young children and that the majority of children with NF1-PN who need treatment, will need to stay on drug for a relatively long period of time, posing significant challenges in terms of long-term tolerability, safety and, last but not least sustainability for the health system and/or other reimbursement mechanisms.

Early data on response after re-challenge at the same time, suggest that it is also possible, after a planned period of time (2–3 years), to consider a “drug holiday” based on clinician, or parent’s shared decision, with the back-up option to restart MEKi in case of rebound growth after treatment interruption [23].

The role of MEKi against atypical Neurofibroma (AN/ANNUBP) is still unclear but some cases may still respond while on treatment. However, it seems also clear from SPRINT and other dataset that MEKi cannot prevent the malignant degeneration of PN to a MPNST. Therefore, any PN which progress while on MEKi should raise the suspicion of an ongoing degeneration whose additional somatic mutations (CDKN2A, PRC, TP53) render the treatment ineffective [45].

1.5 Conclusions

The treatment paradigm of PN has dramatically changed since the use of MEKi, which proved able to alter the natural growth trajectory of PN in children and, in many cases, a significant short-term clinical benefit.

Long-term side effects, overall benefit as well as optimization of treatment indication, duration and tolerability represent key unanswered questions which need to be addressed.

Upcoming collaborative projects (Eu-Pearl) are in the pipelines paving the way towards a more patient-centered approach to identify and prospectively validate PRO/ObsRO measures that specifically assess PN-related morbidities focusing on QOL as a first important step to significantly ameliorate and mitigate PN morbidities.

2. Surgical management of neurofibromatosis type

2.1 The plastic surgery contributes to therapeutic neurofibroma treatment

The distinctive tumor of NF1 is the neurofibroma. Histologically, neurofibromas are tumors that develop from peripheral nerves and are made up of a variety of cell types, including Schwann cells, myelinated and unmyelinated axons, fibroblasts, endothelial cells, and mast cells [46]. Discrete cutaneous neurofibromas develop at dermal nerve terminals. They present as soft, well-defined, sessile or pedunculated nodules with clinical findings that range in size from a few millimeters to several centimeters. Although stinging and itching sensations can be annoying, they rarely cause pain or discomfort. Subcutaneous neurofibromas are firm rubbery nodules that arise along the course of the peripheral nerve beneath the dermis and they can be painful and tender.

Numerous lesions, even thousands, appear primarily on the face, trunk, and proximal limbs.

Malignant transformation in these tumors is rare although the emotional and social impact can affect a patient's quality of life [47, 48]. Plexiform neurofibromas represent a significant cause of patient morbidity. Plexiform neurofibromas occur in approximately 30–50% of patients who have NF1.

They are composed of the same cell types as cutaneous neurofibromas [49]. Massive tumors known as diffuse plexiform neurofibromas spread to nearby organs, bones, and soft tissues. A deep tumor may be indicated by thicker and hyperpigmented skin that is overlaying the area. Plexiform neurofibromas can develop within the first year of life or be present at birth in patients with neurofibromatosis, with a frequency of 24,1–32%. These tumors' size and location affect how clinically significant they are. They may show up as painful lesions under the skin or asymptomatic bumps. They have the ability to fill space and produce a mass impact when close to significant structures because of their growing potential.

They are also related to a 10% risk of malignant degeneration. The progression tendency of these neurofibromas cannot be established a priori, however, associated risk factors have been identified. Head and neck localization, age < 10 years, and incomplete surgical excision are in fact associated with an increased progression rate [27, 47].

Malignant Peripheral Nerve Sheath Tumors are quite rare in the general population, with an incidence of 0.001%. However, as many as 60% occur in patients with N1, with an approximately 10% lifetime risk of developing it. These are highly aggressive tumors that usually evolve from plexiform neurofibromas. In NF1-affected patients, they generally have an earlier onset, around the second and third decades of life, and a worse prognosis [47, 50]. Unfortunately, surgery is still the only available therapeutic option for this type of neurofibroma because it is impossible to forecast how it will develop over time.

The time and type of surgery are the two most challenging considerations about surgical treatment. Large neurofibromas can require subtotal surgical resection, which may require a staged procedure (**Figures 1** and **2**).

According to our experience, early radical surgery during the initial procedure will result in the greatest long-term outcomes. Each patient must receive individualized care, taking into account the needs that are dictated by their particular diseases. A multidisciplinary approach is the best form of care for people with neurofibromatosis,

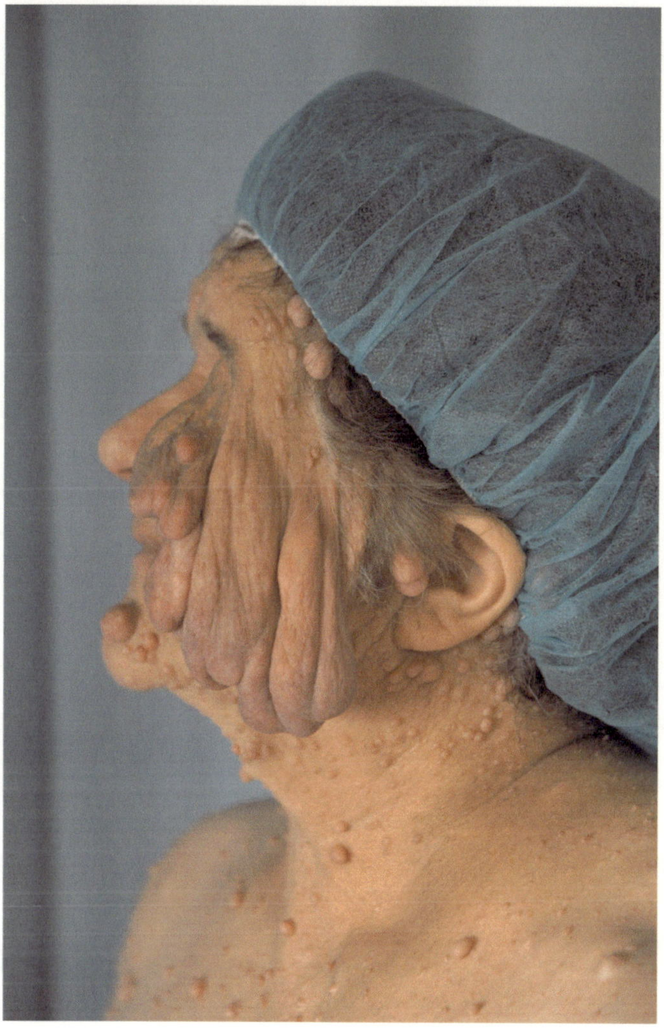

Figure 1.
Voluminous plexiform neurofibroma of the upper eyelid in patient with NF1.

both in children and adults. Each patient is different and presents particular difficulties for the patient's healthcare professionals. Making timely and suitable judgments requires knowledge of the disease, how it progresses, and any potential morbidities. Timing of the operation will depend on symptoms, deformities, disability, and disease development.

Surgery as the last choice is frequently not the most effective option and can produce more severe morbidity. A well-timed operation can significantly reduce long-term deformity and impairment.

The surgical approach of cutaneous and subcutaneous neurofibromas is generally simpler. Since the extension is limited to the epidermal-dermal level, pre-operative imaging investigations are generally not required. The surgery goal is not only to radically remove the lesion but to ensure an aesthetical outcome. The type of reconstruction depends both on the size and the excision area. Minor excisions without skin

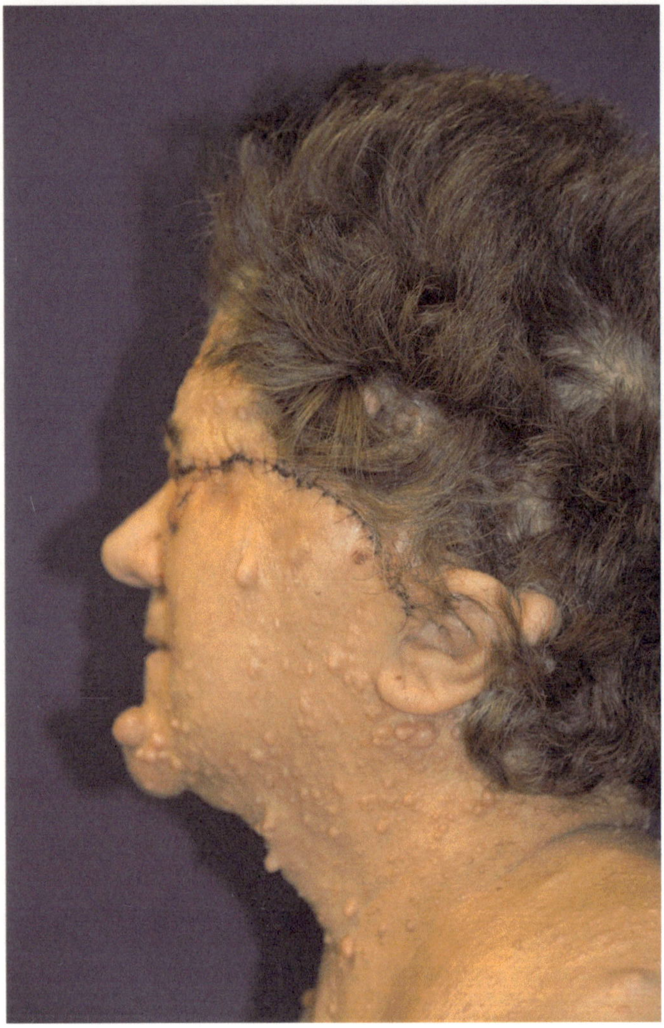

Figure 2.
One-week follow-up after neurofibroma removal and eyelid reconstruction surgery.

tension can be addressed with direct sutures. Following the surgical ladder, major lesions on the other hand may require graft usage, collecting the donor skin from a neurofibromas-free area, and local, pedunculated or free flaps.

The NF1-affected patient will often present with multiple neurofibromas to be removed. In cases of multiple modest-size cutaneous neurofibromas, a considerable number of lesions can be removed within the same surgical session. The limit of removable lesions under local anesthesia depends on the amount of anesthetic that can be safely used, and on the patient's tolerance. In our experience, it is not rare to reach a dozen removed neurofibromas per single surgical session (**Figure 3**). To avoid misunderstandings and exaggerated expectations, however, a priority of the lesions being removed should be agreed upon with the patient before the surgery, leaving any others for future sessions.

Likewise, especially for neurofibromas involving high esthetic interest areas, such as the face, it is advisable to make sure that the patient understands that he will have a

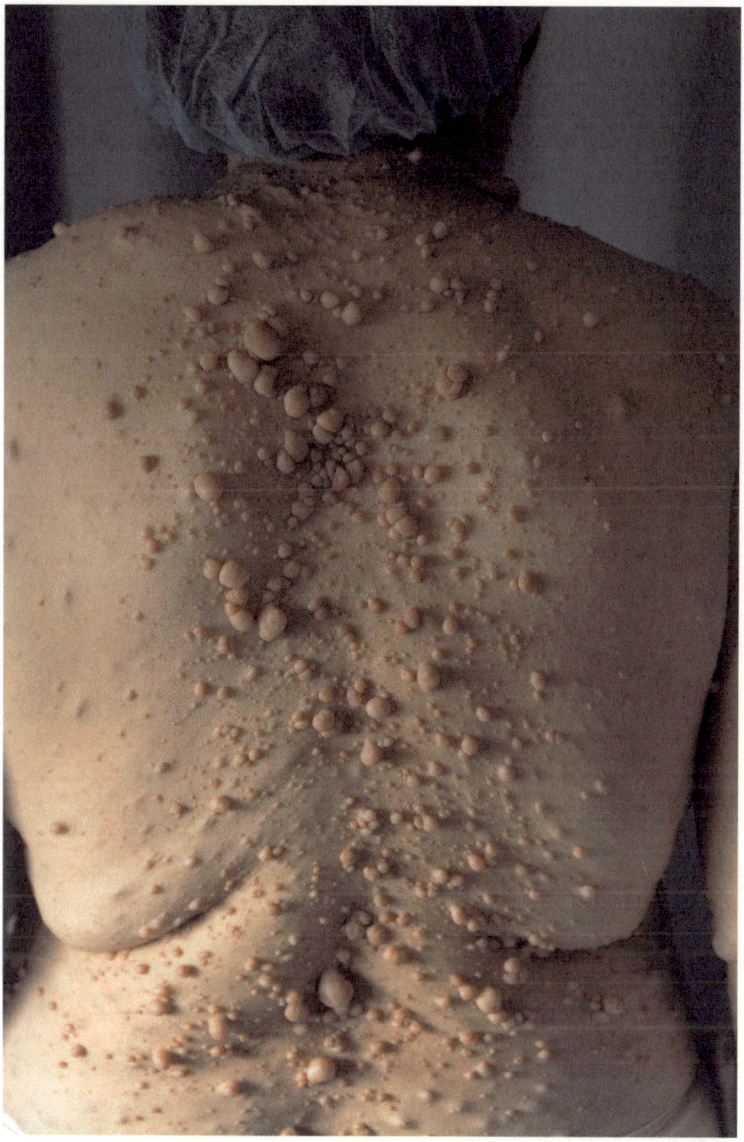

Figure 3.
Numerous cutaneous neurofibromas in patient with NF1.

scar in place of the neoformation. Scar massages with silicon-based gels should be recommended for the 2–3 months after surgery, to promote proper scar maturation.

In case of unsatisfactory results, the patient should be invited to wait at least six months or one year before a possible touch-up. Both scars and blemishes can improve over time, making surgery superfluous. The risks relating to these surgeries are rather limited. They mainly concern possible recurrence and surgical wound complications, such as delayed healing, dehiscence, or local infection. No absolute indications for antibiotic therapy are recommended, but if comorbidities that can favor infection onsets are present, the operator may recur to pre-operative antibiotic prophylaxis [51].

The histological examination should always be requested for each excision, even once the diagnosis has already been formulated. Plexiform neurofibromas, on the other hand, represent a tougher surgical challenge. For surgical excision indications, in addition to the esthetic and pain, which they share with cutaneous neurofibromas, they present functional impairment. Following significant volumetric growth, they can compress nerve structures and lead to functional deficits.

A periodic follow-up is the only valid method to monitor their evolution and evaluate surgery indications. Preoperative imaging is required and MRI is considered the gold standard. Compared to other methods such as ultrasound or CT, MRI allows a better margins definition, which is often unclear, a better tissue distinction, and the evaluation of nerve/vascular infiltration and local invasion. MRI can also be used to classify plexiform neurofibromas into three classes: superficial, displacing, and invasive [52].

The excision should be as radical as possible to avoid tumor recurrences.

Early interventions seem to improve both the outcome, as the exeresis operation remains more confined without extending to other districts, and the recurrence rate.

Ideally, the tumor should be removed at its superficial level, as this appears to effectively prevent a recurrence. Once the tumor is in the invasive phase, the recurrence rate is in fact around 20%, rising to 46% for incompletely excised cases [53].

For advanced neoformations, when the tumor grows to invade nerve fascicles, it could be unfeasible for the surgeon to remove it without having to sacrifice the nerve, thus causing a possible functional deficit of which the patient must be informed during the collection of informed consent for surgery.

Among the potential risks, the vascularization status of these neoformations should be investigated during pre-operative routines.

In the case of particularly vascularized neurofibromas, known as hemangioneurofibromas, angiography with pre-operative embolization can be planned, to significantly reduce bleeding risk during and after surgery [54].

Acting as subcutaneous expanders, a skin laxity could remain after these tumors' enucleation. If this happens, a skin lozenge could be removed around the incision to re-tension the tissues.

Especially for large volumes tumors, it is possible, after performing accurate hemostasis, to place a drain to prevent hematomas and seromas formation.

In the case of voluminous neurofibromas involving lower limbs, the possibility of prescribing anticoagulant therapy or the use of elastic stockings until normal walking is resumed is advisable to prevent deep vein thrombosis. Antibiotic prophylaxis may be indicated if there are concurrent risk factors for infection or a drain is in place.

MRI is the reference diagnostic to evaluate the tumor extent and its relationship with adjacent structures. However, to confirm the lesion malignancy, it is necessary to resort to other methods like F-2-deoxy-D-glucose positron emission tomography (FDG-PET), which can also detect the presence of distant metastases. Nevertheless, a biopsy is required for histological confirmation. Since at least 2 centimeters of tumor-free margins are recommended for these lesions, the biopsy can be excisional for lesions smaller than 3–4 cm. For larger lesions, multiple core-needle biopsies, possibly ultrasound or CT-guided, are recommended. Incisional biopsies are less used since they are burdened by a greater complications risk, and are often limited to a single sample collection, albeit of larger dimensions.

Adjuvant radiotherapy may be used to address medium and high-grade lesions. Although it does not improve overall survival, it seems to improve the local management of the tumor. Adjuvant chemotherapy is reserved for systemic metastatic diseases instead [47, 55].

The requirement to perform a wide resection to ensure disease-free margins often results in major nerve sacrifice and consequent functional damage. Although regarded as the last resort, limb amputation may sometimes be necessary to ensure adequate cancer radicalization [56].

Complications are similar to those resulting from the enucleation of large plexiform neurofibroma. Nonetheless, the patient should be informed about the bad prognosis and the high recurrence rate of these tumors. Tumors bigger than 5 centimeters, local invasiveness, distant metastases, and non-radical surgery are all negative prognostic factors [57].

The 5-year local recurrence rate ranges from 27–49%. Distant metastases are instead reported between 26–65%, and mainly involve the lungs, brain, skeletal system, and liver [58].

Because of this high recurrence rate, careful follow-up is mandatory. Clinical evaluations should be performed every three months for the first two years, and an imaging investigation is recommended at least twice a year.

2.2 Role of neurosurgery in the treatment of nerve tumors in patients with neurofibromatosis type 1

The treatment of nerve tumors in patients with NF1 is multidisciplinary; it involves geneticists, oncologists, neurosurgeons and plastic surgeons mainly.

Surgery is in all cases reserved for symptomatic lesions or malignant evolution; the neurosurgeon is involved in lesions of nerve plexuses and trunks or in case of extension of the pathology within the spinal canal with resultant myelopathy.

Special attention and a dedicated experience in the treatment of these lesions is essential as the functioning nerve fascicles in these lesions are incorporated in the tumor and may not always be dissected from it. This surgery is potentially at risk of increasing additional neurological deficits and the extent of the removal must be limited to what is necessary.

2.2.1 Neurofibroma

Neurofibromas can be located in any peripheral nerve or root; they originate from Schwann cells and grow in the nerve by dividing the nerve fibers without infiltrating them; due to this characteristic, it is generally possible to remove them without determining a reduction in neurological function as they only require the sacrifice of the usually non-functioning original fiber. On the contrary, neurofibromas and plexiform neurofibromas (PNs) are complex conglomerates of intraneural neurofibromas that create tortuous and huge masses arising in nerve trunks (**Figures 4** and 5). PNs are pathognomonic and typical manifestation of NF1 (30% patients with NF1 have clinical evident PNs; with RM study incidence grows to 50–60%) [23], potentially involving almost every part of the body outside of the brain and spinal cord. They can also occur on the face (including around the eyes), neck, arms, legs, back, chest, abdomen, and internal organs. Large tumors cause the nerves (also superficial sensory nerves) to become thick and misshapen, which can affect the structure of nearby bone, skin, and muscle. Especially large and deforming PNs can cause severe pain, mobility problems, vision and hearing loss, high blood pressure and other medical problems. They commonly occur in children and most of them are not cancer, but some may later become cancer. When present on major nerve trunks they involve multiple fascicles.

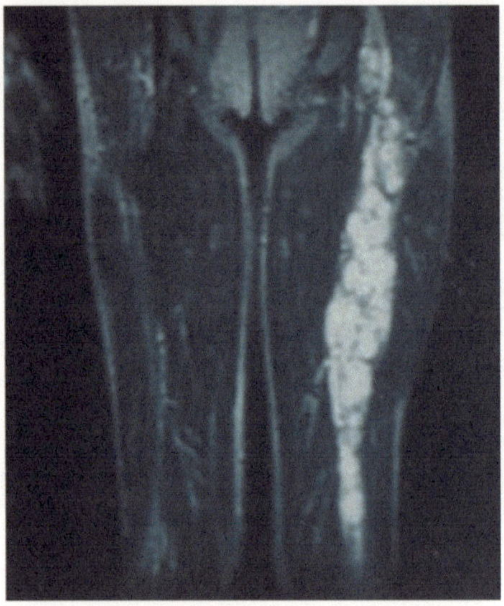

Figure 4.
MRI imaging of plexiform neurofibroma of left sciatic nerve.

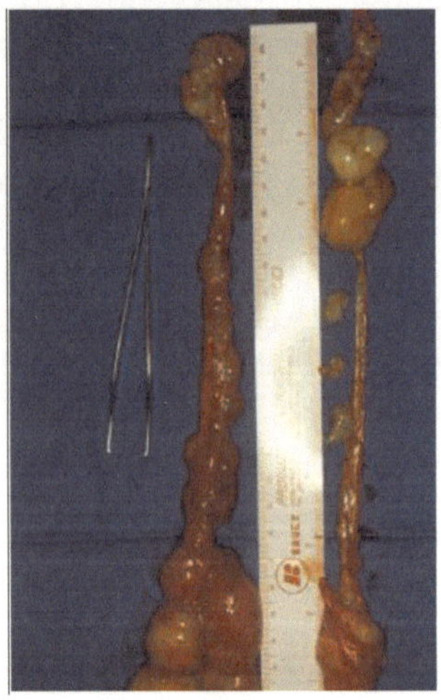

Figure 5.
Left sciatic plexiform neurofibroma after surgical removal.

Therefore, the removal of such lesions can lead to sensorimotor deficits, including neuropathic pain, in patients that can develop in the future other lesions. This kind of surgery to be safely performed requires experience and expertise in this field. For all the above-mentioned reasons surgery in cases of NPs is limited to lesions with suspected malignant degeneration or resulting in neurological deficits although, not infrequently some patients ask for the removal of large PNs also for esthetic and functional problems.

MPNSTs are the malignant variant of peripheral nerve tumors; although they also originate from Schwann cells, due to their aggressive behavior, they are mostly considered as sarcomas. These lesions, that are very rare in the general population, have a high incidence among patients with NF1 and are one of the most frequent causes of death in patients with this disease [59]. The chance of a patient with NF1 developing an MPNST is estimated to be between 8 and 15% [2]. Among NF1 patients with a microdeletion, this percentage rises to 16–26% [59]. The 5-year overall survival between patients with MPNST is about 20–50% [12] with a worst outcome in metastatic or unresectable lesions; actually, the survival in the population with NF1 is like similar to the general one. This progress in related to a better follow up and an early diagnosis in patients with NF1.

2.2.2 Indications for surgery

The indication for surgery for nerve tumors in patients with NF1 is limited to cases symptomatic of neurological deficits or suspected malignancy of the mass. Since there is growing evidence that MEK inhibitors may play a significant role in their treatment (of PNs). The risks of surgery needs to be balanced against the possibility to offer a conservative management based on pharmacological treatments now available for selected cases [59, 60]. This is especially true for those large disfiguring multi-embryonic derivation PNs (affecting nerves, cartilage, bone and dermis) where the surgical results leave much to be desired. However, considering the period of several weeks required for the medical treatment to show the first results, it is straight forward that for the following conditions, a drug treatment approach cannot be the solution.

2.3 Malignancy

The lifetime chance of developing a malignancy (MPNST) in a NF1 patient is reportedly 8–15%; at least in 1/3 of cases, they arise from PNs and bulky masses (≥6 cm) seem predisposed to turn malignant. The factors that may favor malignancy are not known except a previous radiation treatment [23]. Clinical signs of a malignant evolution are rapid growth, spontaneous sharp pain and neurological deficit of the affected nerve. The growth of a neurofibroma is a common event especially in children and adolescents in which the masses often grow consensually with physical development; on the other hand, it is unusual to have a significant growth in adults, in whom a volumetric increase greater than 20% per year represents an important index of suspicion [23]. Currently, patients with NF1 undergo periodic clinical and instrumental checks in specialized centers to identify early clinical or radiological manifestations of possible malignant evolution. This is to ensure prompt diagnosis and treatment. An early diagnosis, in fact, can significantly improve the life prognosis. Sometimes the MPNST arises de novo but, in most cases, it is a progressive degeneration of a nodule within plexiform neurofibromas that accumulate genetic alterations becoming atypical neurofibromatous neoplasm of uncertain biological potential (ANNUBP), lesions with potential malignant evolution. From the anatomopathological point of view, this entity, also defined as atypical neurofibroma, is gaining importance. This lesion, which from the radiological and clinical point of view seems to be indistinguishable from a benign one, presents histological features (atypia, loss of neurofibroma architecture, high cellularity and/or mitotic activity between 1:50 and 3:10 high power fields) that are similar to MPNST and seems to be a precursor of malignant nerve sheath tumors [12, 61]. The use of PET CT with fludeoxyglucose (FDG) and volumetric MRI [62] can precociously identify lesions harboring these characteristics, so allowing their complete removal if the mass is easily reachable, or a diagnostic biopsy if the tumor is placed in less accessible sites. In detail,

PET CT is capable of early identification of masses undergoing malignant transformation, as they have a more active metabolism; however, this type of investigation has a better sensitivity but rather low specificity since there is a non-negligible overlapping of uptake values between lesions undergoing a malignant evolution and lesions that are still benign [12, 23, 62, 63]. The removal in the case of MPNST must be aggressive, sacrificing the nerve of origin regardless of its function. Radicality with free surgical margins must be obtained and this is of paramount importance; if the lesion, on the other hand, is an ANNUBP, the removal can be confined to the tumor without the extension beyond its margins. Therefore, an early diagnosis not only improves the prognosis, but also allows avoidance of destructive interventions if it is not the case.

2.4 Neurological deficits

Neurinomas, neurofibromas and PNs generally are benign lesions, and they do not cause neurological deficits; neurological deficits appear either because they cause compression on the spinal cord having an intracanal growth or because the nerve itself becomes deficient as the tumor grows within an anatomical bottleneck.

2.4.1 Spinal cord compression

Spinal cord compression from root neurinomas or neurofibromas represents an important clinical problem in patients with NF1; it generally occurs at the cervical or at lumbosacral level due to an intracanal growth of huge NFS of brachial and lumbar plexus. Patients develop progressive quadriparesis or paraparesis, incontinence and spinal pain. The objective of the surgery is the decompression of the spinal cord which is obtained not only through the removal of the mass (in the case of a neurinoma) but also through a decompressive hemilaminectomy and a large dural plastic. Performing a widening of the spinal canal during the surgical procedure ensures that even a possible regrowth of the neurofibroma is better tolerated by the patient and does not interfere with neurological integrity. These surgical procedures generally lead to a regression of spinal compression symptoms [64–68], but the removal of root lesions can cause a major sensory damage to the nerves involved. The recurrence of pyramidal symptoms is rare since normally the growth of even these intracanal lesions tends to slow down with increasing age.

2.4.2 Nerve deficits

Diffuse enlargement of all major peripheral nerve trunks occurs in some individuals with particularly aggressive forms of NF1 due to the development of multiple plexiform neurofibromas, isolated neurofibromas, and schwannoma [68, 69]. When examined, these subjects often present partial deficits of peripheral nerves which have arisen slowly and progressively and of which often the patients are unaware. We are dealing with deficits affecting nerves that grow into anatomical bottlenecks such as the olecranon canal, Froehse's arcade or the peroneal arch at the head of the fibula; the growth of any neoplasm within an anatomical narrowing may cause deficit of the nerve trunk itself and pain. The treatment of this type of problem consists of removing all or part of the tumor mass to reduce the volume of the nerve along with decompression at the physiological anatomical narrowing. While widening the anatomical narrowing appears to be a safe maneuver, the removal of the NPs in an already deficient nerve is not risk-free and must be carefully evaluated. This type of procedure mostly serves to prevent a further worsening of the deficit and must be performed only at the request of the patient. The worsening of these deficits is slow and progressive, sometimes accompanied by modest pain; from this point of view it clearly differs from the growth of malignancies which, on the contrary, appear sudden and extremely painful.

2.5 Aesthetical reasons

At light of the new therapeutic proposals, an attempt with the so-called RAS therapy (selumetinib is in a phase II trial) is in our opinion always worth to be firstly attempted.

We have witnessed some astonishing results especially in those cases where the aesthetical problem seems to be prevalent. Surgery, when a complex malformation of the superficial layers is involved, where the dermis and the convoluted superficial nerves often infiltrate and deform the underlying muscles, very rarely attains a satisfactory result.

3. Surgery

3.1 General consideration

According to these guidelines, surgery is performed. The patients are usually under general anesthesia in the absence of curare or in spinal anesthesia; magnified vision with microscope or loupes is required; the exposure of the tumor must be adequate with the possibility of identifying both the nerve entering and exiting the mass. This is easily obtained in limb lesions, while in large masses in deep sites, this type of exposure may be difficult to achieve [59]. Once exposed, the mass is inspected under a microscope and mapped to identify the eloquent nerve bundles that need to be spared. The tumor capsule should be opened in the direction of the fibers in areas silent to stimulation and then the main tumor nodules and their fibers of origin should be identified. The possibility of radical removal is linked to the specific histology of the lesion.

3.2 Neurinomas

Neurinomas of peripheral nerves practically always appear to be radically removable as the tumor grows by dividing the nerve fibers which are distributed on the surface of its capsule. An intracapsular removal of the mass allows a complete and safe en bloc removal, leaving the nerve fibers intact on the capsule left in place. An intracapsular removal is currently accepted and recognized as safe; moreover, it is absolutely not associated with a risk of recurrence (**Figures 6** and 7).

An exception is represented by cystic schwannomas, a very insidious subgroup as a surgical outcome. In fact, in neurinomas with these characteristics, the thin wall of the tumor mass does not always seem recognizable concerning the capsule. In an attempt to remove it altogether, sometimes, part of the capsular wall is removed, damaging the fibers contained therein, thus creating a neurological deficit. For this reason, in cystic neurinomas, it is sometimes advisable to subtotal excision and emptying of the cyst to avoid nerve damage.

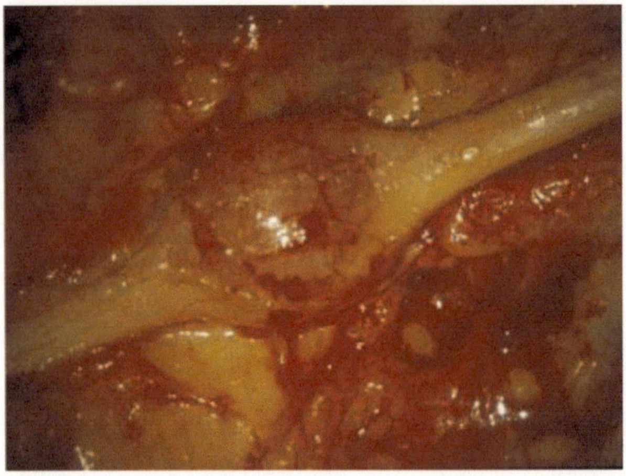

Figure 6.
Surgical appearance of a neurinoma.

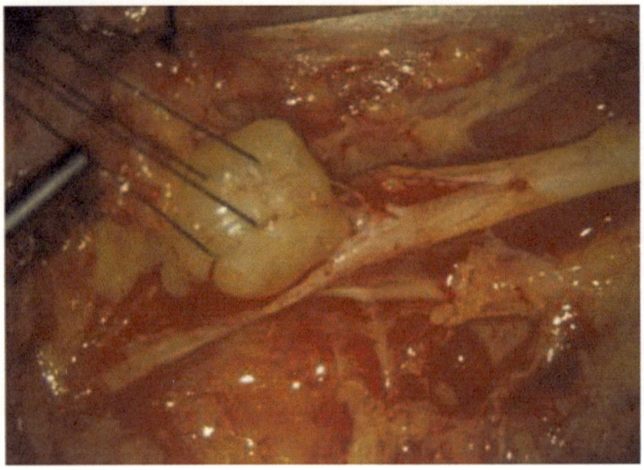

Figure 7.
Removal of a neurinoma: Surgical technique.

3.3 Neurofibromas and plexiform Neurofibromas

Neurofibroma and plexiform neurofibroma appears as fusiform and multiple enlargements of the nerve and the fibers appear dispersed within the neoplasm (**Figures 8–10**).

Sometimes the removal of the nodules in plurinodular neoplasms entails the sacrifice of some fascicles conducting when stimulated. In this case it is necessary to carefully evaluate the contribution of each fascicle to the general function of the nerve and limit the removal to the most voluminous or suspicious nodules, at times preparing for a subtotal debulking to avoid neurological deficits [70]. In fact, the functioning fascicles can be sometimes the origin of the neoplasm and appear inseparable from the rest of the tumor: therefore, an accurate balance with direct stimulation or with the use of NAPs (nerve action potentials) is mandatory [59]. The surgical treatment of these lesions challenges the surgeon's ability to approach localized masses in every part of the body and sometimes in deep thoracic, abdominal or pelvic areas for which an

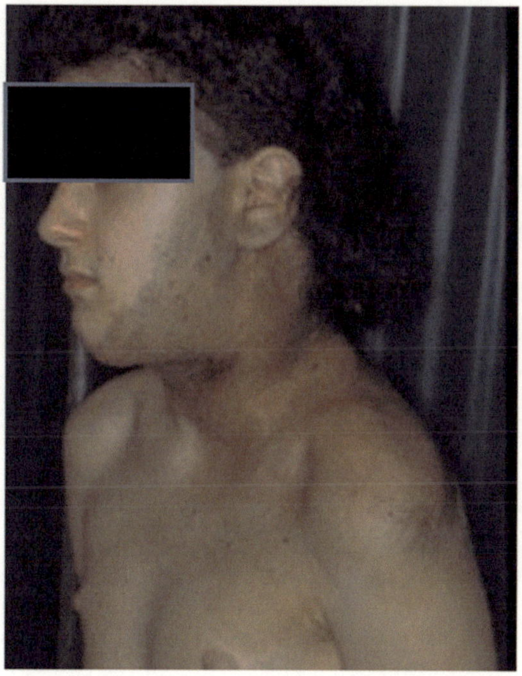

Figure 8.
Clinical appearance of plexiform neurofibroma of the neck involving brachial plexus.

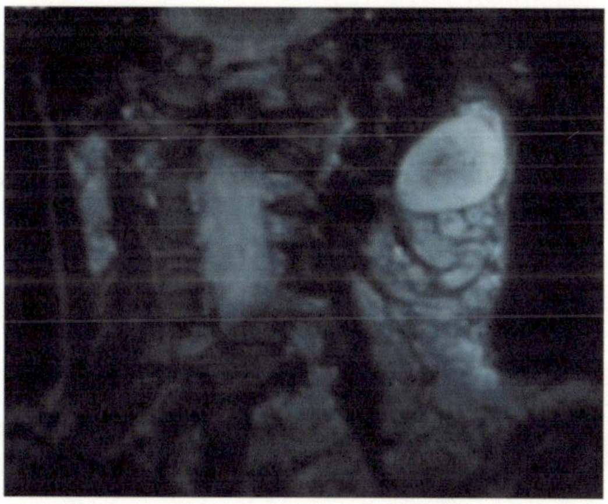

Figure 9.
Its radiological appearance.

anatomical knowledge of these regions may not be straightforward. A basic expertise of general or urologic surgery is often required coupled with experience in the field of nerve surgery. It is important to be able to remove the lesion in the desired way already at the first surgical procedure; having to re-operate on nerve tumors in which there has been previous manipulation with consequent development of scar tissue, makes it much more difficult and significantly increases the risk of post-surgical neurological deficits. The first surgery is the best possibility we have to obtain a total removal: this must be the mantra. Therefore, the best possible removal must be

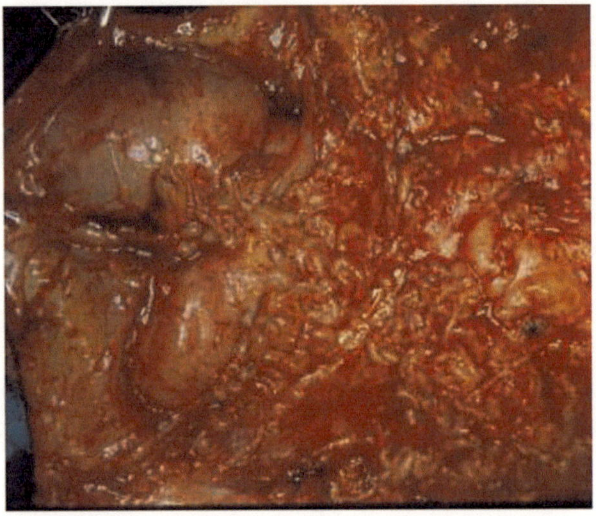

Figure 10.
Intraoperative imagine of plexiform neurofibroma of the neck involving brachial plexus.

accurately planned since the very first observation of the case. In addition to the risk of causing neurological deficits, the removal of large plexiform neurofibromas involving large parts of the body and skin can cause massive blood loss with acute hypovolemia and significant post-operative hematomas in the surgical cavity.

3.4 MPNST, ANNUBP and atypical neurofibromas

Particular attention is required for the surgical technique to be used in case of suspected or proven malignancy of the mass. Even more, in this situation, wide exposure of the lesion is necessary.

In the case of atypical neurofibromas or ANNUBP, the mass is often asymptomatic and morphologically identical to a benign neurofibroma. Surgery only requires the complete removal of the mass without the need to sacrifice the nerve in its entirety. The removal may be restricted to the fascicle of origin as the malignant component is inside the nodule [12, 59]. While orthodoxy, in the case of MPNST, dictates a complete removal with margins free from disease (**Figure 11**), the possibility of saving part of the nerve of origin, that is not involved in the neoplasm, should be considered only for small lesions and to safeguard very delicate functions (es. ulnar of median intrinsic function of the hand) where the nerve cannot be easily repaired or replaced with a nerve transfer technique.

The patient should be informed in advance and eventually accept the risk of a local recurrence, with the possibility of reintervention in the short term and, theoretically, the occurrence of distant metastases. Obviously, the patient will undergo close follow-up to detect an early recurrence of the illness. In the experience of our department, the use of this surgical technique has not been affected by an increase in mortality and morbidity; on the contrary, it was possible to preserve the nervous function without worsening the prognosis and with only one out of eight patient who needed reoperation. Complete healing was obtained after the second surgery. The attitude towards those cases of MPNST coming to attention in an advanced stage and

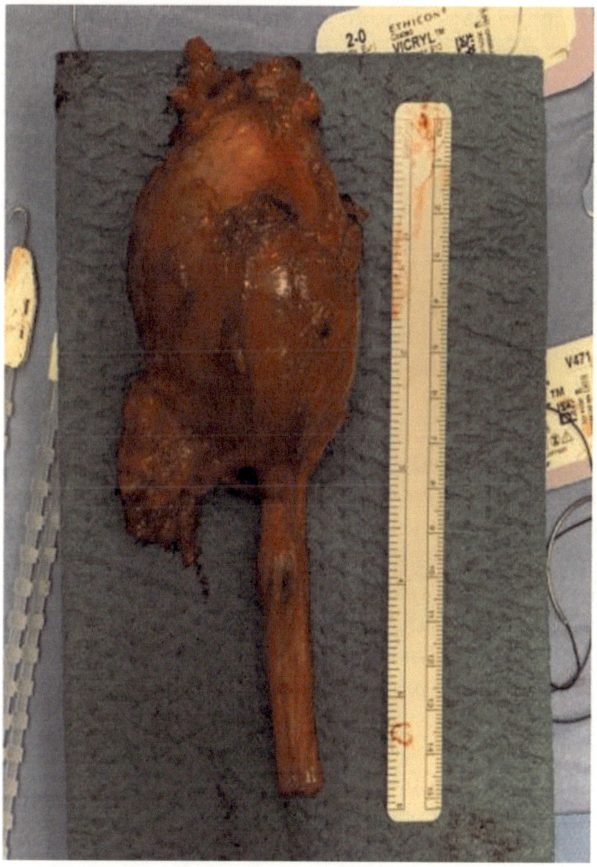

Figure 11.
Sciatic MPNST removed with sacrifice of the nerve.

originating from the lumbar or lumbosacral plexus is completely different; often the lesions are large (>10 cm) and have engulfed arteries and veins.

Accurate staging of the disease is necessary before proceeding with surgery. In the surgical approach it is important to consider the relationship and the tumor infiltration of the vessels which must be investigated previously with angiography or angioCT. If there is arterial or venous encasement, the main vessels must be prepared upstream and downstream of the lesion both to control bleeding and to proceed with a vascular bypass if the vessel cannot be sacrificed. Once more, every effort is made to obtain a complete removal of the mass and radicality as much as possible. Unfortunately, experience has demonstrated that when a malignant lesion presents these characteristics, despite excellent surgical treatment, the prognosis is in any case poor; the only result is a prolongation of survival. On the other hand, surgery currently appears to be the only valid treatment available in the case of MPNST; conventional radiotherapy, hadron therapy (proton beam seems to be more effective) and chemotherapy treatments have very poor results in slowing the progression of the disease and have no curative chance. This underlines the importance of early diagnosis of MPNST, to detect the disease as long as it appears surgically removable in a radical way [61, 70, 71]. Individuals with NF1 appear to be the population at greatest risk for this pathology. The attending physicians and specialists who treat such patients with

NF1 must be vigilant and pay attention to signs and symptoms that may herald the onset of this pathology for a prompt diagnosis.

3.5 Reconstructive technique

In the event of a destructive surgery such as required by MPNSTs or in the unfortunate exceptions of neurological deficits following the removal of neurofibromas and neurinomas, the surgeon must be able to schedule reconstructive or secondary surgery to guarantee the patient the best possible quality of life. Patients with NF1 present specific problems as it is not always easy to respect one of the basic concepts of nerve surgery, that the sutured nerves must be completely healthy; an anatomical classical repair would involve suturing nerve stumps that are not completely tumor-free.

Therefore, the first choice in these injuries, if technically possible, is palliative surgery. This consists in surgical muscle transfer techniques which act by modifying the insertions and levers of the muscles spared from injury. The new tendon insertions change their effect and restore lost functions. Examples of such techniques are the posterior tibialis muscle transfer in case of foot drop due to common peroneal nerve palsy or the triple transfer according to Merle d'Aubignè to restore wrist and finger dorsiflexion in the event of a radial nerve injury [72]. These techniques also have the advantage of giving an almost immediate result as they do not need to wait for the natural regrowth of the nerve. In very extensive lesions such as in cases of MPNST of the brachial or lumbosacral plexus, it may be necessary to apply reconstructive techniques following the same principles as in traumatic nerve or plexus injuries [72]. In fact, when possible, nerve transfers are an even better alternative to muscle transfers, since they ensure a natural reinnervation of the lost muscles. First-choice techniques are the direct reinnervations of distally sectioned nerves; They do not require grafts nor nerve sutures in surgical site where radiotherapy will or could be performed. For example, in complete injuries of the brachial plexus, multiple extraplexual reinnervation can be used, such as an accessory-suprascapular nerve for the shoulder and intercostal to muscolocutaneous nerve to recover the bicipital function [73]. The site of repair is so completely outside the region to be irradiated and a good chance of nerve repair is assured.

4. Illustrative cases

4.1 Case 1

An 18-year-old woman with NF1 due to a de novo variant was referred to our department after a 6 month of sharp right arm pain, right brachial plexus palsy and a rapidly growing bulky supraclavicular mass. On physical examination, the patient presented an initial tetraparesis and the MRI of the right brachial plexus showed a voluminous supraclavicular and infraclavicular mass lesion involving the entire brachial plexus, with encasement of the subclavian artery and vein and intracanal extension at the level of C7 with radiological signs of cervical myelopathy (**Figures 12** and **13**). The investigations clearly suggested a diagnosis of MPNST. Staging performed showed no further localization of disease. After an angio-CT study of the vessels, the patient underwent surgery to remove the mass in two stages. In the first stage, the patient underwent right C4-T1 hemilaminectomy with the aid of sensory

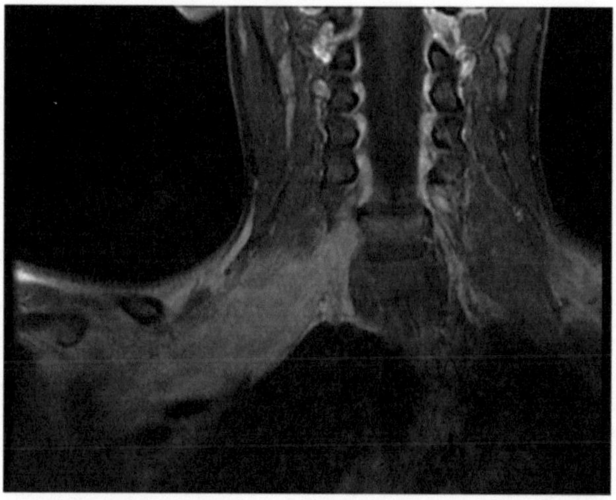

Figure 12.
MR imaging of a right brachial plexus MPNST.

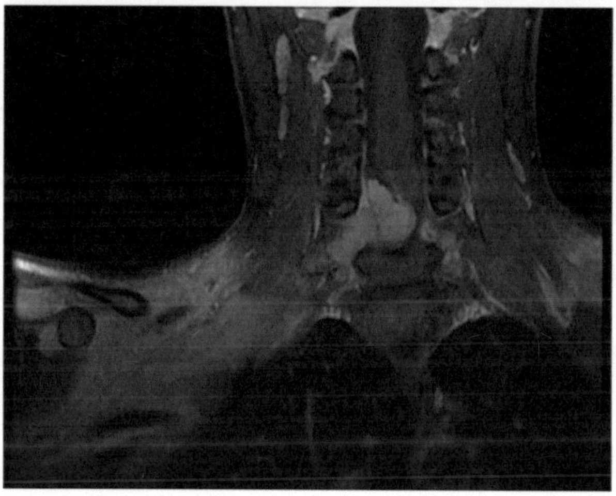

Figure 13.
MR imaging of a right brachial plexus MPNST.

and motor evoked potential monitoring and removal of the intracanal component of the lesion. The posterior roots of C7 from which the tumor originated were highlighted (**Figure 14**); they were isolated and detached from the spinal cord and the intracanal component was completely removed (**Figure 15**). Dural plasty and closure of the dura of the C7 foramen was performed. The second approach consisted of a large anterior exposure with removal of the right half of the sternal manubrium and 2/3 of the clavicle without disarticulating the sternoclavicular joint; the subclavian vessels have been exposed up to their origin from the anonymous trunks (**Figure 16**). The tumor was isolated by sectioning the roots at the entrance and the nerves at the exit; the vessels were freed from the neoplasm and their walls did not appear to be infiltrated, therefore bypass was not performed. At the end of the procedure, the removal appeared macroscopically complete. In the same session, an accessory suprascapular reinnervation was performed with a view to a future reconstruction as

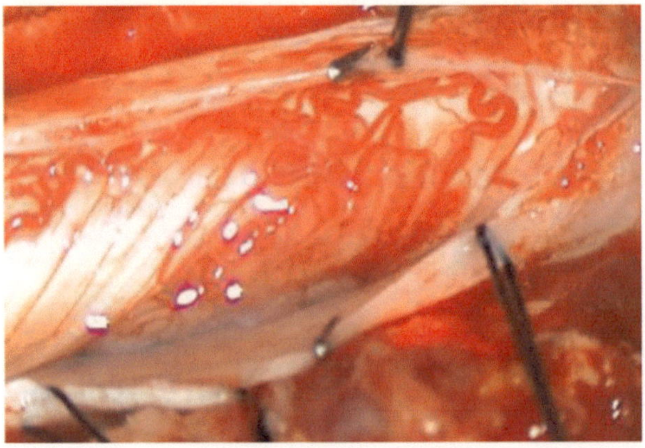

Figure 14.
C7 root with MPNST infiltration.

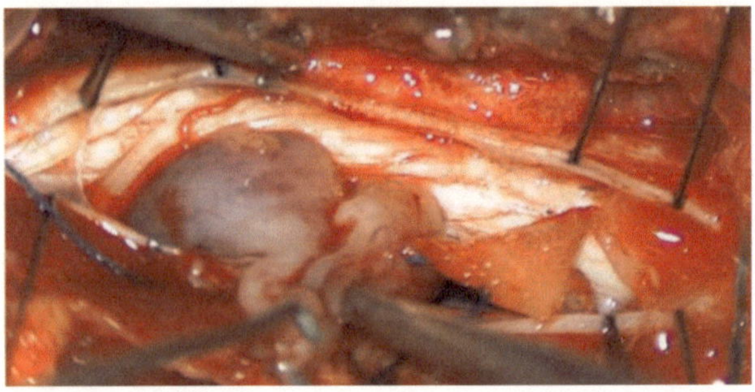

Figure 15.
Removal of intradural extension of MPNST.

the suture would have been outside the radiotherapy treatment field. Subsequently, in case of a good survival, reinnervation of the musculocutaneous would have been planned with intercostals and a gracilis free flap to recover some function of the hand. The patient was referred for radiotherapy treatment on the surgical focus. Unfortunately, 8 months after surgery, a dissemination of disease was observed in the intradural spinal area: no further surgical options were possible, and the patient was referred for oncological treatment.

4.2 Case 2

A 14-year-old girl with NF1 was referred to our department for evaluation of a rapidly growing mass in a previously known plexiform neurofibroma of the femoral region of the right leg. The patient did not present any pain or neurological deficit but the rapid evolution of the lesion and its MR appearance gave evidence for a possible malignant evolution (**Figures 17** and **18**). Surgical removal was planned. The removal of the mass was radical with the possibility of preserving most of the fibers of the femoral nerve (**Figure 19**); the patient did not present any neurological deficit.

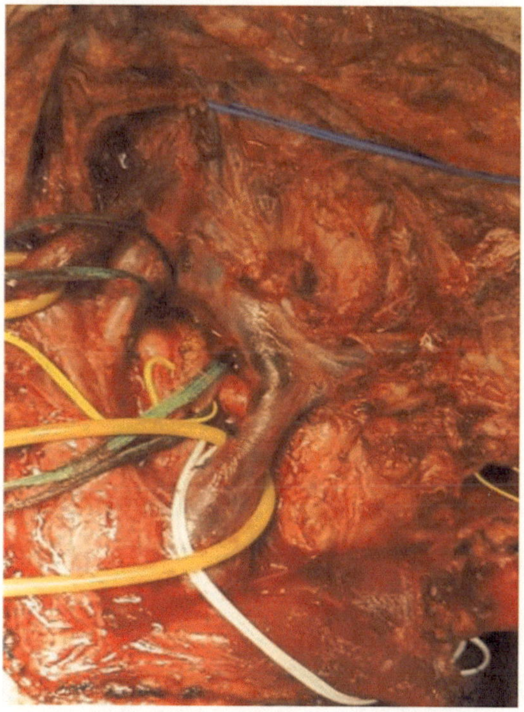

Figure 16.
Anterior approach with exposition of subclavian vessels encased in the MPNST.

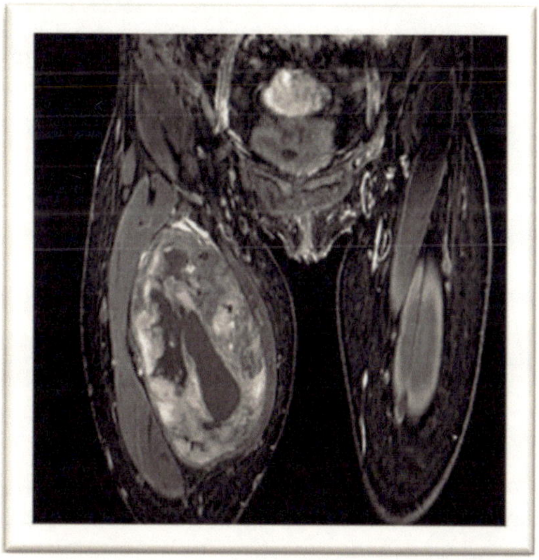

Figure 17.
MR appearance of a low grade MPNST of right femoral nerve.

Histological examination indicated an atypical neurofibroma with foci of malignancy. After the surgical procedure, the patient with a follow-up of more than 5 years did not present any disease recurrence.

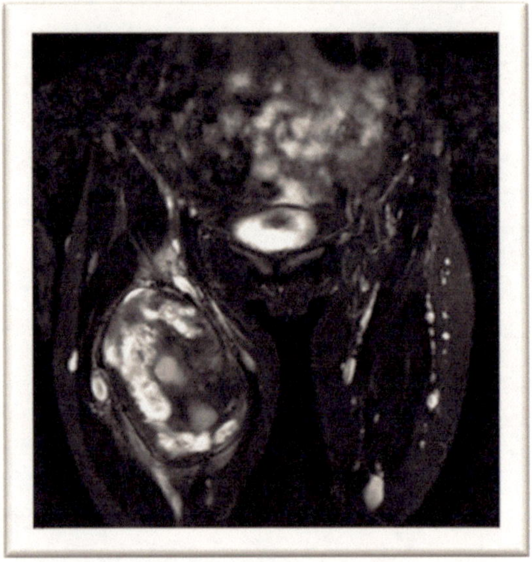

Figure 18.
MR appearance of a low grade MPNST of right femoral nerve.

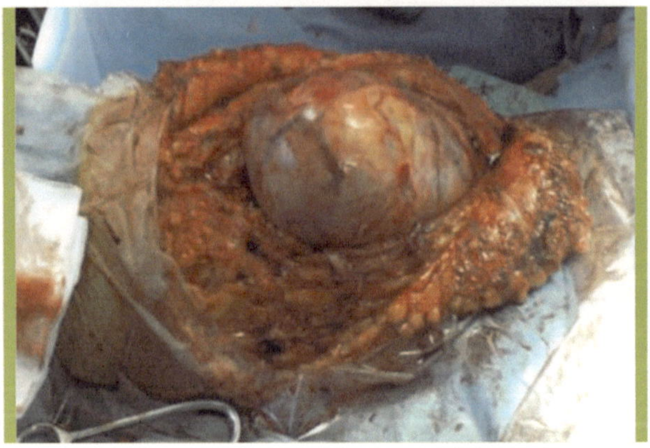

Figure 19.
Low grade MPNST of the femoral nerve; intraoperative image.

5. Conclusion

The treatment of peripheral nerve tumors in patients with NF1 appears complex when these lesions develop in the main nerve trunks and the plexuses; nevertheless, there are some general principles to respect:

Surgery is not definitively curative; therefore, it must be limited to severely symptomatic lesions or when a possible malignant evolution is dreaded.

Neurinomas are generally removable without damage and radically; however, it is advisable to pay attention to the predominantly cystic forms, whose total removal can often be achieved at the expense of a nerve lesion.

In the case of PNs, despite the present indication that medical therapy is only when a mass is declared inoperable, we think that apart from cases where malignancy is suspected or an immediate result is expected (such as spinal cord compression), surgery must stay in a second plane.

It is necessary to evaluate and limit the removal of the PNs not to worsen the patient's condition with post-surgical neurological deficits.

Any lesion rapidly growing, severely painful, and that causes neurological deficits should be considered suspicious for MPNST until proven otherwise.

All patients with NF1 should undergo periodic check-ups to detect lesions with potential malignant evolution in a very early phase and treat them promptly.

For all the above considerations, the patient affected by NF1 needs to be followed and treated by a highly specialized multidisciplinary team that can offer all the treatments and therapies available at the state-of-the-art.

6. Future directions and developments in NF1-PN research

6.1 Extracellular matrix and tumor development: a new therapeutic scenario

NF1 is caused by a pathogenic variant in the NF1 tumor suppressor gene, which is located at chromosome 17q11.2.5 In 90% of the cases, the mutation leads to a loss of function of the NF1 gene product neurofibromin type I (Nf1, comprising 2818 residues, UniProt: P21359–2) [74]. This giant protein (320 kDa) is a GTPase-activating protein promoting the conversion of active guanosine triphosphate (GTP)-bound RAS to its inactive guanosine diphosphate (GDP)-bound conformation [8]. Unexpected layers of regulation for biological regulation Nf1 have been opened by recent studies on cryo-Electron microscopy (cryo-EM). Nf1 works as a dimeric architecture resting in an equilibrium between open and close conformational states (including an auto-inhibited closed conformation [75]. The structure derives from a dynamic interaction of known Nf1 domains as the GAP-related domain (GRD), the phosphatidylinositol-transfer protein Sec14p-homologous domain, and the Pleckstrin-homology domain module, together referred to as Sec14-PH domain. The GRD carries out Ras GAP activity and interacts via its GAP-extra domain (GAPex) with SPRED proteins [76]. Remarkably, genetic variants within these regions have been linked to NF1 or Legius syndromes, proposing the importance of all domains for neurofibromin function [77].

The GRD is locked down into a crevice formed by the alpha-helical repeat scaffold by an interprotomer interaction. The GAPex domain is formed by residues flanking the GAP core. Strikingly, in this position, the GRD-binding site for Ras is occluded by the surrounding CDM, suggesting that the observed neurofibromin conformation does not represent its active state.

Moreover, Nf1 can directly bind glycerophospholipids and phosphoinositide lipids on the plasma membrane through the Sec14-PH domain and the C-terminal Sprouty domain of SPRED proteins [78, 79]. These data account for functional interaction with the signaling platforms active in cell homeostasis composed of multiple molecules such as tyrosine kinase receptors and their downstream effectors; likewise, they suggest new potential Nf1 plasma membrane targets on the membrane as Src, integrin/Fak complexes.

Haploinsufficiency for Nf1 causes growth factor-dependent hyperactivation of Ras (11), which further increases when loss of heterozygosis (LOH) of NF1 occurs [3]. LOH is considered the primary process behind neurofibromas onset due to the activation of several signaling axes downstream Ras as Raf /ERK, PI3K/AKT, and mTOR in Schwann cells. In addition to its role in the negative regulation of Ras, neurofibromin is a positive regulator of adenylyl cyclase, the enzyme responsible for the generation of intracellular cyclic AMP (cAMP) [4, 80, 81]. This knowledge leads to pharmacologically targeting these upstream and downstream effectors such as growth factor receptors [82, 83] mTOR [30, 84], and MAP Kinase MEK [10]. MEK inhibitors-based treatment is the most successful treatment. Among MEK inhibitors, selumetinib has been recently approved for PNST treatment by the Food and Drug Administration [10, 33]. The partial therapeutic response of MEK inhibitors has been ascribed to the multifaced nature of tumor biology.

As learned from other tumor models, Ras hyperactivation is insufficient per se to promote neoplastic growth and progression: it requires a second hit to promote neoplastic growth. According to the advances in other tumors, cooperation of Ras signaling with biochemical and biophysical signals provided by a heterozygous niche ($NF1^{+/-}$) [4] induces neoplastic transformation of a cell [85]. Accordingly, growing literature states that increasing matrix stiffness generated in abnormal tissues as fibrotic tissues functionally contribute to tumor progression and dissemination through profound modification of the tumor cell genome landscape [85, 86]. Indeed, the main feature of neurofibroma is a potent extracellular matrix (ECM) structure due to the massive deposition of insoluble and soluble proteins by abnormally activated fibroblasts; nevertheless, its role in tumor progression is still poorly defined. Recently, Errico et al. explored whether Ras signaling could be potentiated by ECM-mediated inward signaling. They demonstrated that Focal adhesion Kinase is a crucial enzyme able to integrate and potentiate both ECM-dependent of inward signaling and the Ras/Raf/Erk and PI3K downstream signaling, thus creating a potent tumorigenic axis. Remarkably, combinatorial treatment with the FAK inhibitor defactinib (VS-6063) and selumetinib (AZD6244) selectively suppressed the colony growth of Schwann cells. These data pave the way for a new therapeutic route based on disrupting the ECM-sensing machinery [18]. PNs appear with a serpentine pattern with multiple patchy nodules with thick collagen fibers [87]. In pancreatic ductal adenocarcinoma (PDAC), these fibers, typical of fibrotic tissues, have been shown to potently induce both FAK and RAS family GTP hydrolases (RHO GTPases) activity influencing the genome landscape of the cancer cells.

In general, an abnormal, stiff matrix is generated by active fibroblasts or Fibrosis Associated Fibroblasts (FAF) or myofibroblasts, robustly secreting many of the constituents of the ECM and basement membranes — such as type I, type III, and type IV and type V collagens, laminins and fibronectin and growth factors. Indeed, activated fibroblasts were first described in the setting of wound healing and were recognized predominantly by their ability to form a scar and later to be critical cells in the chronic tissue wound healing response, also known as tissue fibrosis.

In neurofibromas, many myofibroblasts in the stroma implicate their essential role in fibrosis development. However, both the cellular type from which they originate and the local biological process sustaining their transition are still under debate [88]. Parrinello et al. in 2008 have launched the idea that neurofibroma begins from a wound healing process initiated by Nf1 loss sufficient *per se* to affect axon/Schwann cells association and trigger a nerve repair process through Schwann cell dedifferentiation, immuno-cells recruitment, and resident fibroblasts activation [89].

Several pieces of evidence corroborate the hypothesis that neurofibroma resembles a wounded nerve that never heals, although they do not explain the neoplastic progression of Schwann cells: a common feature possessed by Schwann cells and many other cells is the injury-induced activation of genes associated with epithelial–mesenchymal transitions and stemness (see below), differentiation states that are linked to cellular plasticity and that help injury-induced tissue remodeling. PN's Schwann cells coexist in distinct subpopulations of Schwann cells at various differentiation states and remarkable plasticity [90]; Nerve repair depends on myelin dedifferentiation but also on the activation of transcriptional mechanisms that were not necessarily involved in Schwann cell development; two transcriptional controls, c-Jun and chromatin modifications involving H3K27 demethylation, H3K27 deacetylation, and H3K4 methylation, were found to be essential for the normal execution of the Schwann cell injury response. The H3K27 demethylation correlates to tumor progression towards malignancy, since is considered a suitable marker in Atypical Neurofibromatous Neoplasm with Uncertain Biological Potential (ANNUBP) [14]; Choi et al. found that the gene expression profiles of neurofibroma from genetically engineered mouse (Nf1flox/flox; DhhCre, [91]) and rat sciatic nerve, following crush injury were similar [92]; this mouse model, generated neurofibromas with wild type niche, enriched by macrophages; macrophages are critical determinants in Schwann cell reprogramming towards mesenchymal state during peripheral nerve regeneration. However, the macrophage population is poorly represented in human plexiform neurofibromas and scarcely investigated in other mouse models of PN (Nf1flox/flox; Krox20-Cre, [93] Nf1flox/flox; PlpCre [94]; these inflammatory cells, in malignant evolution of PN, the MPNSTs, are significantly characterized suggesting that they do not appear to be necessary for tumorigenesis, but likely contribute to aspects of plexiform neurofibroma progression [95]. By contrast, Nf1-haploinsufficient mast cells are abundantly recruited by stem cell factors (SCFs) secreted by Schwann cells that lack neurofibromin (Nf1−/−). Moreover, compared with normal mast cells, SCF-stimulated heterozygous mast cells (Nf1+/−) secreted 2.5-fold more transforming growth factor beta (TGF-β) [96]. Thus, the direct cooperation of Schwann cells and myofibroblasts generates a continuous mast cell recruitment in the neurofibroma that may explain the onset and maintenance of a chronic inflammation disrupting homeostatic regulation of the wound healing (**Figure 20**).

A self-renewing loop is triggered, since mast cell-derived TGFβ promotes epithelial-mesenchymal transition (EMT)-like changes in fibroblasts and other cell type as pericytes or endothelial cells, that trans-differentiates into highly secreting TGFβ myofibroblasts. TGFβ is a master EMT regulator and wound healing regulator and has been previously linked to peripheral nervous system (PNS) regeneration and wound healing and fibrosis [97]. Schwann cells from PNs consistently harbor phosphorylated Smad3 (p-Smad3), active PI3K, and protein kinases (MAPK), the canonical downstream effectors of the TGFβ pathway. In this view, the paracrine feedback loop of Schwann cell-myofibroblasts-mast cell leads to tumor formation due to the combination of Ras hyperactivity and potent secretion of growth factors in a fibrotic milieu. Similarly, in PDAC, TGFβ is a direct modulator of cancer-Schwann cell interactions. Indeed, Schwann cells, chemoattracted by myofibroblasts, are found to directly enhance the aggressiveness of pancreatic cancer cells by secreting TGFβ through SMAD activation; high levels of TGFβ signaling activation positively correlated with perineural invasion by cancer cells suggesting that TGFβ is an essential supporter of both fibrosis and transforming potential [98]. Imatinib, designed to block tyrosine phosphorylation of Smad4 and restores TGF-β growth-suppressive signaling in BCR-ABL1-positive leukemia, has been tested in a phase 2 clinical trial in a patient with inoperable PNs, given its ability to inhibit also tyrosine activity of Kit and PDGF-β receptors. The main trial outcome was tumor shrinkage. The authors observed in a significant subgroup of patients around 20% of tumor reduction, in a subset of

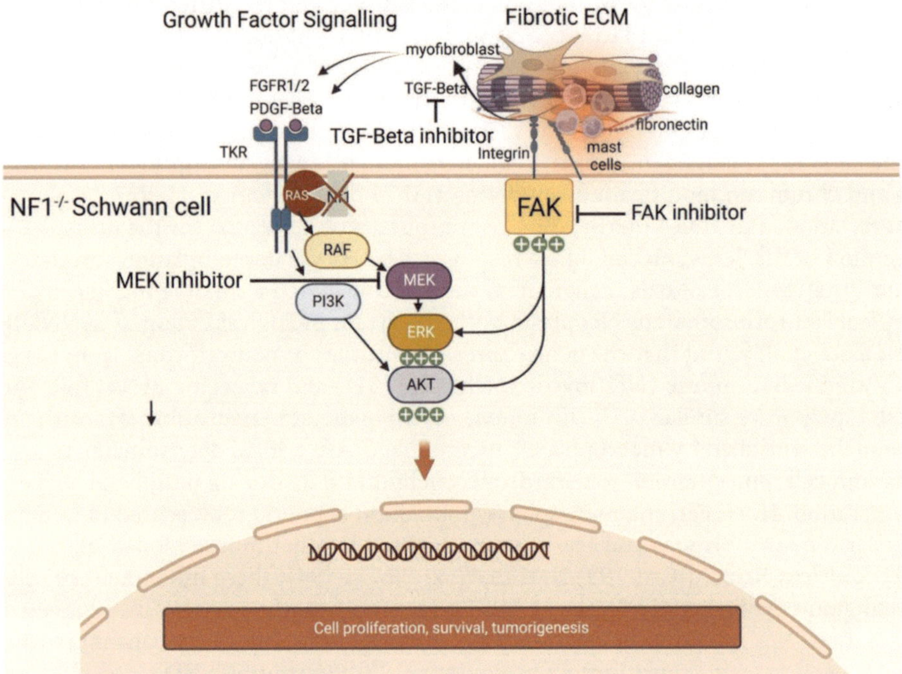

Figure 20.
Ras hyperactivation- and fibrotic extracellular matrix-dependent signaling cooperate to promote tumorigenesis. (Figure made with biorender).

pre-existing PNs. These results suggest that TGF-β inhibitors against SMAD- and non-SMAD downstream signaling must represent an alternative or combinatorial therapeutic solution to MEK inhibitors to achieve therapeutic success [99].

Acknowledgements

We thank all patients for their advice, humanity, and patience, represented by patient Associations such as Linfa OdV https://www.linfaneurofibromatosi.com/.

Conflict of interest

The authors declare no conflict of interest.

Author details

Elisabetta Basso[1*], Enrico Opocher[2], Franco Bassetto[3], Martina Grigatti[3], Alvise Montanari[3], Stefano Ferraresi[1] and Federica Chiara[4*]

1 Department of Neurosurgery, Santa Maria della Misericordia Hospital, Rovigo, Italy

2 Pediatric Hematology, Oncology and Stem Cell Transplant Division, Padua University Hospital, Italy

3 Plastic Surgery Department, Hospital University of Padua, Italy

4 Department of Surgery, Oncology and Gastroenterology, University of Padua, Italy

*Address all correspondence to: federica.chiara@unipd.it; elisabetta.basso@aulss5.veneto.it

IntechOpen

© 2023 The Author(s). Licensee IntechOpen. This chapter is distributed under the terms of the Creative Commons Attribution License (http://creativecommons.org/licenses/by/3.0), which permits unrestricted use, distribution, and reproduction in any medium, provided the original work is properly cited.

References

[1] Legius E, Messiaen L, Wolkenstein P, Pancza P, Avery RA, Berman Y, et al. Revised diagnostic criteria for neurofibromatosis type 1 and Legius syndrome: An international consensus recommendation. Genetics in Medicine. 2021;**23**:1506-1513. DOI: 10.1038/s41436-021-01170-5

[2] Bergqvist C, Servy A, Valeyrie-Allanore L, Ferkal S, Combemale P, Wolkenstein P, et al. Neurofibromatosis 1 French national guidelines based on an extensive literature review since 1966. Orphanet Journal of Rare Diseases. 2020; **15**:37. DOI: 10.1186/s13023-020-1310-3

[3] Harrisingh MC, Lloyd AC. Ras/Raf/ERK signalling and NF1. Cell Cycle. 2004;**3**:1255-1258. DOI: 10.4161/cc.3.10.1182

[4] Gutmann DH, Ferner RE, Listernick RH, Korf BR, Wolters PL, Johnson KJ. Neurofibromatosis type 1. Nature Reviews. Disease Primers. 2017;**3**: 17004. DOI: 10.1038/nrdp.2017.4

[5] Ruggeri RM, Benevento E, De Cicco F, Fazzalari B, Guadagno E, Hasballa I, et al. Neuroendocrine neoplasms in the context of inherited tumor syndromes: A reappraisal focused on targeted therapies. Journal of Endocrinological Investigation. 2023;**46**:213-234. DOI: 10.1007/s40618-022-01905-4

[6] Uusitalo E, Rantanen M, Kallionpaa RA, Poyhonen M, Leppavirta J, Yla-Outinen H, et al. Distinctive cancer associations in patients with Neurofibromatosis type 1. Journal of Clinical Oncology. 2016;**34**: 1978-1986. DOI: 10.1200/JCO.2015.65.3576

[7] Cimino PJ, Ketchum C, Turakulov R, Singh O, Abdullaev Z, Giannini C, et al. Expanded analysis of high-grade astrocytoma with piloid features identifies an epigenetically and clinically distinct subtype associated with neurofibromatosis type 1. Acta Neuropathologica. 2023;**145**:71-82. DOI: 10.1007/s00401-022-02513-5

[8] Cichowski K, Jacks T. NF1 tumor suppressor gene function: Narrowing the GAP. Cell. 2001;**104**:593-604.1

[9] Stucky CC, Johnson KN, Gray RJ, Pockaj BA, Ocal IT, Rose PS, et al. Malignant peripheral nerve sheath tumors (MPNST): The Mayo Clinic experience. Annals of Surgical Oncology. 2012;**19**:878-885. DOI: 10.1245/s10434-011-1978-7

[10] Gross AM, Dombi E, Widemann BC. Current status of MEK inhibitors in the treatment of plexiform neurofibromas. Child's Nervous System. 2020;**36**: 2443-2452. DOI: 10.1007/s00381-020-04731-2

[11] Dombi E, Solomon J, Gillespie AJ, Fox E, Balis FM, Patronas N, et al. NF1 plexiform neurofibroma growth rate by volumetric MRI: Relationship to age and body weight. Neurology. 2007;**68**: 643-647. DOI: 10.1212/01.wnl.0000250332.89420.e6

[12] Miettinen MM, Antonescu CR, Fletcher CDM, Kim A, Lazar AJ, Quezado MM, et al. Histopathologic evaluation of atypical neurofibromatous tumors and their transformation into malignant peripheral nerve sheath tumor in patients with neurofibromatosis 1-a consensus overview. Human Pathology. 2017;**67**:1-10. DOI: 10.1016/j.humpath.2017.05.010

[13] Pemov A, Hansen NF, Sindiri S, Patidar R, Higham CS, Dombi E, et al.

Low mutation burden and frequent loss of CDKN2A/B and SMARCA2, but not PRC2, define premalignant neurofibromatosis type 1-associated atypical neurofibromas. Neuro-Oncology. 2019;**21**:981-992. DOI: 10.1093/neuonc/noz028

[14] Higham CS, Dombi E, Rogiers A, Bhaumik S, Pans S, Connor SEJ, et al. The characteristics of 76 atypical neurofibromas as precursors to neurofibromatosis 1 associated malignant peripheral nerve sheath tumors. Neuro-Oncology. 2018;**20**: 818-825. DOI: 10.1093/neuonc/noy013

[15] Prudner BC, Ball T, Rathore R, Hirbe AC. Diagnosis and management of malignant peripheral nerve sheath tumors: Current practice and future perspectives. Neuro-oncology Advances. 2020;**2**:i40-i49. DOI: 10.1093/noajnl/vdz047

[16] Brohl AS, Kahen E, Yoder SJ, Teer JK, Reed DR. The genomic landscape of malignant peripheral nerve sheath tumors: Diverse drivers of Ras pathway activation. Scientific Reports. 2017;**7**:14992. DOI: 10.1038/s41598-017-15183-1

[17] Staser K, Yang FC, Clapp DW. Pathogenesis of plexiform neurofibroma: Tumor-stromal/hematopoietic interactions in tumor progression. Annual Review of Pathology. 2012;**7**: 469-495. DOI: 10.1146/annurev-pathol-011811-132441

[18] Errico A, Stocco A, Riccardi VM, Gambalunga A, Bassetto F, Grigatti M, et al. Neurofibromin deficiency and extracellular matrix cooperate to increase transforming potential through FAK-dependent signaling. Cancers (Basel). 2021;**13**:2329. DOI: 10.3390/cancers13102329

[19] Le LQ, Parada LF. Tumor microenvironment and neurofibromatosis type I: Connecting the GAPs. Oncogene. 2007;**26**:4609-4616. DOI: 10.1038/sj.onc.1210261

[20] Akshintala S, Baldwin A, Liewehr DJ, Goodwin A, Blakeley JO, Gross AM, et al. Longitudinal evaluation of peripheral nerve sheath tumors in neurofibromatosis type 1: Growth analysis of plexiform neurofibromas and distinct nodular lesions. Neuro-Oncology. 2020;**22**:1368-1378. DOI: 10.1093/neuonc/noaa053

[21] Plotkin SR, Bredella MA, Cai W, Kassarjian A, Harris GJ, Esparza S, et al. Quantitative assessment of whole-body tumor burden in adult patients with neurofibromatosis. PLoS One. 2012;**7**: e35711. DOI: 10.1371/journal.pone.0035711

[22] Dombi E, Baldwin A, Marcus LJ, Fisher MJ, Weiss B, Kim A, et al. Activity of Selumetinib in Neurofibromatosis type 1-related plexiform Neurofibromas. The New England Journal of Medicine. 2016;**375**:2550-2560. DOI: 10.1056/NEJMoa1605943

[23] Fisher MJ, Blakeley JO, Weiss BD, Dombi E, Ahlawat S, Akshintala S, et al. Management of neurofibromatosis type 1-associated plexiform neurofibromas. Neuro-Oncology. 2022;**24**:1827-1844. DOI: 10.1093/neuonc/noac146

[24] Guha D, Davidson B, Nadi M, Alotaibi NM, Fehlings MG, Gentili F, et al. Management of peripheral nerve sheath tumors: 17 years of experience at Toronto Western hospital. Journal of Neurosurgery. 2018;**128**:1226-1234. DOI: 10.3171/2017.1.JNS162292

[25] Yoshinaga A, Tsuge I, Yoshinaga D, Ogino S, Sakamoto M, Saito S, et al. Reduction of intraoperative bleeding in

diffuse plexiform Neurofibroma resection using the LigaSure vessel sealing system. Plastic and Reconstructive Surgery. 2021;**148**:344e-346e. DOI: 10.1097/PRS.0000000000008163

[26] Canavese F, Krajbich JI. Resection of plexiform neurofibromas in children with neurofibromatosis type 1. Journal of Pediatric Orthopedics. 2011;**31**:303-311. DOI: 10.1097/BPO.0b013e31820cad77

[27] Needle MN, Cnaan A, Dattilo J, Chatten J, Phillips PC, Shochat S, et al. Prognostic signs in the surgical management of plexiform neurofibroma: The Children's Hospital of Philadelphia experience, 1974-1994. The Journal of Pediatrics. 1997;**131**:678-682. DOI: 10.1016/s0022-3476(97)70092-1

[28] Ikuta K, Nishida Y, Sakai T, Koike H, Ito K, Urakawa H, et al. Surgical treatment and complications of deep-seated nodular plexiform Neurofibromas associated with Neurofibromatosis type 1. Journal of Clinical Medicine. 2022;**11**: 5695. DOI: 10.3390/jcm11195695

[29] Robertson KA, Nalepa G, Yang FC, Bowers DC, Ho CY, Hutchins GD, et al. Imatinib mesylate for plexiform neurofibromas in patients with neurofibromatosis type 1: A phase 2 trial. The Lancet Oncology. 2012;**13**:1218-1224. DOI: 10.1016/S1470-2045(12)70414-X

[30] Weiss B, Widemann BC, Wolters P, Dombi E, Vinks A, Cantor A, et al. Sirolimus for progressive neurofibromatosis type 1-associated plexiform neurofibromas: A neurofibromatosis clinical trials consortium phase II study. Neuro-Oncology. 2015;**17**:596-603. DOI: 10.1093/neuonc/nou235

[31] Jakacki RI, Dombi E, Potter DM, Goldman S, Allen JC, Pollack IF, et al. Phase I trial of pegylated interferon-alpha-2b in young patients with plexiform neurofibromas. Neurology. 2011;**76**:265-272. DOI: 10.1212/WNL.0b013e318207b031

[32] Gross A, Bishop R, Widemann BC. Selumetinib in plexiform Neurofibromas. The New England Journal of Medicine. 2017;**376**:1195. DOI: 10.1056/NEJMc1701029

[33] Gross AM, Wolters PL, Dombi E, Baldwin A, Whitcomb P, Fisher MJ, et al. Selumetinib in children with inoperable plexiform Neurofibromas. The New England Journal of Medicine. 2020;**382**: 1430-1442. DOI: 10.1056/NEJMoa1912735

[34] Gross AM, Glassberg B, Wolters PL, Dombi E, Baldwin A, Fisher MJ, et al. Selumetinib in children with neurofibromatosis type 1 and asymptomatic inoperable plexiform neurofibroma at risk for developing tumor-related morbidity. Neuro-Oncology. 2022;**24**:1978-1988. DOI: 10.1093/neuonc/noac109

[35] Espirito Santo V, Passos J, Nzwalo H, Carvalho I, Santos F, Martins C, et al. Selumetinib for plexiform neurofibromas in neurofibromatosis type 1: A single-institution experience. Journal of Neuro-Oncology. 2020;**147**: 459-463. DOI: 10.1007/s11060-020-03443-6

[36] Cacchione A, Fabozzi F, Carai A, Colafati GS, Baldo GD, Rossi S, et al. Safety and efficacy of Mek inhibitors in the treatment of plexiform Neurofibromas: A retrospective study. Cancer Control. 2023;**30**. DOI: 10.1177/10732748221144930

[37] Baldo F, Grasso AG, Cortellazzo Wiel L, Maestro A, Trojniak MP, Murru FM, et al. Selumetinib in the

treatment of symptomatic intractable plexiform Neurofibromas in Neurofibromatosis type 1: A prospective case series with emphasis on side effects. Paediatric Drugs. 2020;**22**:417-423. DOI: 10.1007/s40272-020-00399-y

[38] Ronsley R, Hounjet CD, Cheng S, Rassekh SR, Duncan WJ, Dunham C, et al. Trametinib therapy for children with neurofibromatosis type 1 and life-threatening plexiform neurofibroma or treatment-refractory low-grade glioma. Cancer Medicine. 2021;**10**:3556-3564. DOI: 10.1002/cam4.3910

[39] Guerreiro Stucklin AS, Mueller S. Opportunities for the treatment of NF1-associated low-grade gliomas: How to decide on the best treatment options for patients? Neuro-Oncology. 2020;**22**: 1415-1416. DOI: 10.1093/neuonc/noaa201

[40] Weiss BD, Wolters PL, Plotkin SR, Widemann BC, Tonsgard JH, Blakeley J, et al. NF106: A Neurofibromatosis clinical trials consortium phase II trial of the MEK inhibitor Mirdametinib (PD-0325901) in adolescents and adults with NF1-related plexiform Neurofibromas. Journal of Clinical Oncology. 2021;**39**:797-806. DOI: 10.1200/JCO.20.02220

[41] Fisher MJ, Shih CS, Rhodes SD, Armstrong AE, Wolters PL, Dombi E, et al. Cabozantinib for neurofibromatosis type 1-related plexiform neurofibromas: A phase 2 trial. Nature Medicine. 2021;**27**:165-173. DOI: 10.1038/s41591-020-01193-6

[42] Klesse LJ, Jordan JT, Radtke HB, Rosser T, Schorry E, Ullrich N, et al. The use of MEK inhibitors in Neurofibromatosis type 1-associated tumors and Management of Toxicities. The Oncologist. 2020;**25**:e1109-e1116. DOI: 10.1634/theoncologist.2020-0069

[43] de Blank P, Fouladi M, Huse JT. Molecular markers and targeted therapy in pediatric low-grade glioma. Journal of Neuro-Oncology. 2020;**150**:5-15. DOI: 10.1007/s11060-020-03529-1

[44] Hanzlik E, Archambault B, El-Dairi M, Schroeder K, Patel MP, Lipp ES, et al. Use of Trametinib in children and young adults with progressive low-grade glioma and Glioneuronal tumors. Journal of Pediatric Hematology/Oncology. 2022;**45**:464-470. DOI: 10.1097/MPH.0000000000002598

[45] Somatilaka BN, Sadek A, McKay RM, Le LQ. Malignant peripheral nerve sheath tumor: Models, biology, and translation. Oncogene. 2022;**41**: 2405-2421. DOI: 10.1038/s41388-022-02290-1

[46] Kimura M, Kamata Y, Matsumoto K, Takaya H. Electron microscopical study on the tumor of von Recklinghausen's neurofibromatosis. Acta Pathologica Japonica. 1974;**24**:79-91. DOI: 10.1111/j.1440-1827.1974.tb00809.x

[47] Parsons CM, Canter RJ, Khatri VP. Surgical management of neurofibromatosis. Surgical Oncology Clinics of North America. 2009;**18**: 175-196. DOI: 10.1016/j.soc.2008.08.009

[48] Wolkenstein P, Zeller J, Revuz J, Ecosse E, Leplege A. Quality-of-life impairment in neurofibromatosis type 1: A cross-sectional study of 128 cases. Archives of Dermatology. 2001;**137**: 1421-1425. DOI: 10.1001/archderm.137.11.1421

[49] Huson SM, Harper PS, Compston DA. Von Recklinghausen neurofibromatosis. A clinical and population study in south-East Wales. Brain. 1988;**111**(Pt 6):1355-1381. DOI: 10.1093/brain/111.6.1355

[50] Grobmyer SR, Reith JD, Shahlaee A, Bush CH, Hochwald SN. Malignant peripheral nerve sheath tumor: Molecular pathogenesis and current management considerations. Journal of Surgical Oncology. 2008;**97**:340-349. DOI: 10.1002/jso.20971

[51] Brambullo T, Biffoli B, Scortecci L, Messana F, Vindigni V, Bassetto F. Antibiotic prophylaxis in plastic surgery: From systematic review to operative algorithm. World Journal of Plastic Surgery. 2022;**11**:24-36. DOI: 10.52547/wjps.11.2.24

[52] Friedrich RE, Korf B, Funsterer C, Mautner VF. Growth type of plexiform neurofibromas in NF1 determined on magnetic resonance images. Anticancer Research. 2003;**23**:949-952

[53] Korf BR. Malignancy in neurofibromatosis type 1. The Oncologist. 2000;**5**:477-485. DOI: 10.1634/theoncologist.5-6-477

[54] Littlewood AH, Stilwell JH. The vascular features of plexiform neurofibroma with some observations on the importance of pre-operative angiography and the value of pre-operative intra-arterial embolisation. British Journal of Plastic Surgery. 1983;**36**:501-506. DOI: 10.1016/0007-1226(83)90140-6

[55] Santoro A, Tursz T, Mouridsen H, Verweij J, Steward W, Somers R, et al. Doxorubicin versus CYVADIC versus doxorubicin plus ifosfamide in first-line treatment of advanced soft tissue sarcomas: A randomized study of the European Organization for Research and Treatment of cancer soft tissue and bone sarcoma group. Journal of Clinical Oncology. 1995;**13**:1537-1545. DOI: 10.1200/JCO.1995.13.7.1537

[56] Vauthey JN, Woodruff JM, Brennan MF. Extremity malignant peripheral nerve sheath tumors (neurogenic sarcomas): A 10-year experience. Annals of Surgical Oncology. 1995;**2**:126-131. DOI: 10.1007/BF02303627

[57] Hruban RH, Shiu MH, Senie RT, Woodruff JM. Malignant peripheral nerve sheath tumors of the buttock and lower extremity. A study of 43 cases. Cancer. 1990;**66**:1253-1265. DOI: 10.1002/1097-0142(19900915)66:6<1253::aid-cncr2820660627>3.0.co;2-r

[58] Anghileri M, Miceli R, Fiore M, Mariani L, Ferrari A, Mussi C, et al. Malignant peripheral nerve sheath tumors: Prognostic factors and survival in a series of patients treated at a single institution. Cancer. 2006;**107**:1065-1074. DOI: 10.1002/cncr.22098

[59] Garozzo D. Peripheral nerve tumors in neurofibromatosis 1: An overview on management and indications for surgical treatment in our experience. Neurology India. 2019;**67**:S38-S44. DOI: 10.4103/0028-3886.250697

[60] Marjanska A, Galazka P, Wysocki M, Styczynski J. New Frontiers in therapy of peripheral nerve sheath tumors in patients with Neurofibromatosis type 1: Latest evidence and clinical implications. Anticancer Research. 2020;**40**:1817-1831. DOI: 10.21873/anticanres.14136

[61] Reilly KM, Kim A, Blakely J, Ferner RE, Gutmann DH, Legius E, et al. Neurofibromatosis type 1-associated MPNST state of the science: Outlining a research agenda for the future. Journal of the National Cancer Institute. 2017;**109**:djx124. DOI: 10.1093/jnci/djx124

[62] Ahlawat S, Fayad LM, Khan MS, Bredella MA, Harris GJ, Evans DG, et al.

Current whole-body MRI applications in the neurofibromatoses: NF1, NF2, and schwannomatosis. Neurology. 2016;**87**: S31-S39. DOI: 10.1212/ WNL.0000000000002929

[63] Valeyrie-Allanore L, Ismaili N, Bastuji-Garin S, Zeller J, Wechsler J, Revuz J, et al. Symptoms associated with malignancy of peripheral nerve sheath tumours: A retrospective study of 69 patients with neurofibromatosis 1. The British Journal of Dermatology. 2005; **153**:79-82. DOI: 10.1111/ j.1365-2133.2005.06558.x

[64] Lavrador JP, Lascelles K, Ferner R, Thomas N, Zebian B. Neurofibroma of the cervical spine in infants. Child's Nervous System. 2016; **32**:2277-2279. DOI: 10.1007/s00381-016-3253-5

[65] van Sandick JW, van Coevorden F. Plexiform neurofibroma with intraspinal extension. Journal of the American College of Surgeons. 2002;**195**:572. DOI: 10.1016/s1072-7515(02)01299-1

[66] Leonard JR, Ferner RE, Thomas N, Gutmann DH. Cervical cord compression from plexiform neurofibromas in neurofibromatosis 1. Journal of Neurology, Neurosurgery, and Psychiatry. 2007;**78**:1404-1406. DOI: 10.1136/jnnp.2007.121509

[67] Wang T, Yin H, Han S, Yang X, Wang J, Huang Q, et al. Malignant peripheral nerve sheath tumor (MPNST) in the spine: A retrospective analysis of clinical and molecular prognostic factors. Journal of Neuro-Oncology. 2015;**122**: 349-355. DOI: 10.1007/s11060-015-1721-5

[68] Pollack IF, Colak A, Fitz C, Wiener E, Moreland M, Mulvihill JJ. Surgical management of spinal cord compression from plexiform neurofibromas in patients with neurofibromatosis 1. Neurosurgery. 1998;**43**:248-255; discussion 255-246. DOI: 10.1097/00006123-199808000-00038

[69] Nguyen R, Kluwe L, Fuensterer C, Kentsch M, Friedrich RE, Mautner VF. Plexiform neurofibromas in children with neurofibromatosis type 1: Frequency and associated clinical deficits. The Journal of Pediatrics. 2011; **159**(652–655):e652. DOI: 10.1016/j. jpeds.2011.04.008

[70] Ross AL, Panthaki Z, Levi AD. Surgical management of a giant plexiform neurofibroma of the lower extremity. World Neurosurgery. 2011; **75**:754-757. DOI: 10.1016/j.wneu.2010. 09.030

[71] Kim A, Stewart DR, Reilly KM, Viskochil D, Miettinen MM, Widemann BC. Malignant peripheral nerve sheath tumors state of the science: Leveraging clinical and biological insights into effective therapies. Sarcoma. 2017;**2017**:7429697. DOI: 10.1155/2017/7429697

[72] Sobczuk P, Teterycz P, Czarnecka AM, Switaj T, Kosela-Paterczyk H, Kozak K, et al. Malignant peripheral nerve sheath tumors - outcomes and prognostic factors based on the reference center experience. Surgical Oncology. 2020;**35**:276-284. DOI: 10.1016/j.suronc.2020.09.011

[73] Kruft S, von Heimburg D, Reill P. Treatment of irreversible lesion of the radial nerve by tendon transfer: Indication and long-term results of the merle d'Aubigne procedure. Plastic and Reconstructive Surgery. 1997;**100**: 610-616; discussion 617-618. DOI: 10.1097/00006534-199709000-00010

[74] Friedman JM. Epidemiology of neurofibromatosis type 1. American Journal of Medical Genetics. 1999;**89**:1-6

[75] Chaker-Margot M, Werten S, Dunzendorfer-Matt T, Lechner S, Ruepp A, Scheffzek K, et al. Structural basis of activation of the tumor suppressor protein neurofibromin. Molecular Cell. 2022;**82**(1288–1296): e1285. DOI: 10.1016/j.molcel.2022.03.011

[76] Dunzendorfer-Matt T, Mercado EL, Maly K, McCormick F, Scheffzek K. The neurofibromin recruitment factor Spred1 binds to the GAP related domain without affecting Ras inactivation. Proceedings of the National Academy of Sciences of the United States of America. 2016;**113**:7497-7502. DOI: 10.1073/pnas.1607298113

[77] Ko JM, Sohn YB, Jeong SY, Kim HJ, Messiaen LM. Mutation spectrum of NF1 and clinical characteristics in 78 Korean patients with neurofibromatosis type 1. Pediatric Neurology. 2013;**48**:447-453. DOI: 10.1016/j.pediatrneurol.2013.02.004

[78] Welti S, Fraterman S, D'Angelo I, Wilm M, Scheffzek K. The sec14 homology module of neurofibromin binds cellular glycerophospholipids: Mass spectrometry and structure of a lipid complex. Journal of Molecular Biology. 2007;**366**:551-562. DOI: 10.1016/j.jmb.2006.11.055

[79] Stowe IB, Mercado EL, Stowe TR, Bell EL, Oses-Prieto JA, Hernandez H, et al. A shared molecular mechanism underlies the human rasopathies Legius syndrome and Neurofibromatosis-1. Genes & Development. 2012;**26**: 1421-1426. DOI: 10.1101/gad.190876.112

[80] Ferner RE. The neurofibromatoses. Practical Neurology. 2010;**10**:82-93. DOI: 10.1136/jnnp.2010.206532

[81] Gutmann DH, Blakeley JO, Korf BR, Packer RJ. Optimizing biologically targeted clinical trials for neurofibromatosis. Expert Opinion on Investigational Drugs. 2013;**22**:443-462. DOI: 10.1517/13543784.2013.772979

[82] Kim A, Dombi E, Tepas K, Fox E, Martin S, Wolters P, et al. Phase I trial and pharmacokinetic study of sorafenib in children with neurofibromatosis type I and plexiform neurofibromas. Pediatric Blood & Cancer. 2013;**60**:396-401. DOI: 10.1002/pbc.24281

[83] Kim A, Lu Y, Okuno SH, Reinke D, Maertens O, Perentesis J, et al. Targeting refractory sarcomas and malignant peripheral nerve sheath tumors in a phase I/II study of Sirolimus in combination with Ganetespib (SARC023). Sarcoma. 2020;**2020**: 5784876. DOI: 10.1155/2020/5784876

[84] Parker VER, Keppler-Noreuil KM, Faivre L, Luu M, Oden NL, De Silva L, et al. Safety and efficacy of low-dose sirolimus in the PIK3CA-related overgrowth spectrum. Genetics in Medicine. 2019;**21**:1189-1198. DOI: 10.1038/s41436-018-0297-9

[85] Laklai H, Miroshnikova YA, Pickup MW, Collisson EA, Kim GE, Barrett AS, et al. Genotype tunes pancreatic ductal adenocarcinoma tissue tension to induce matricellular fibrosis and tumor progression. Nature Medicine. 2016;**22**:497-505. DOI: 10.1038/nm.4082

[86] Yamauchi M, Barker TH, Gibbons DL, Kurie JM. The fibrotic tumor stroma. The Journal of Clinical Investigation. 2018;**128**:16-25. DOI: 10.1172/JCI93554

[87] Messersmith L, Krauland K. Neurofibroma. Treasure Island (FL): StatPearls; 2023

[88] Jiang C, McKay RM, Le LQ. Tumorigenesis in neurofibromatosis type 1: Role of the microenvironment. Oncogene. 2021;**40**:5781-5787. DOI: 10.1038/s41388-021-01979-z

[89] Parrinello S, Noon LA, Harrisingh MC, Wingfield Digby P, Rosenberg LH, Cremona CA, et al. NF1 loss disrupts Schwann cell-axonal interactions: A novel role for semaphorin 4F. Genes & Development. 2008;**22**: 3335-3348. DOI: 10.1101/gad.490608

[90] Mazuelas H, Magallon-Lorenz M, Fernandez-Rodriguez J, Uriarte-Arrazola I, Richaud-Patin Y, Terribas E, et al. Modeling iPSC-derived human neurofibroma-like tumors in mice uncovers the heterogeneity of Schwann cells within plexiform neurofibromas. Cell Reports. 2022;**38**:110385. DOI: 10.1016/j.celrep.2022.110385

[91] Wu J, Williams JP, Rizvi TA, Kordich JJ, Witte D, Meijer D, et al. Plexiform and dermal neurofibromas and pigmentation are caused by Nf1 loss in desert hedgehog-expressing cells. Cancer Cell. 2008;**13**:105-116. DOI: 10.1016/j.ccr.2007.12.027

[92] Choi K, Komurov K, Fletcher JS, Jousma E, Cancelas JA, Wu J, et al. An inflammatory gene signature distinguishes neurofibroma Schwann cells and macrophages from cells in the normal peripheral nervous system. Scientific Reports. 2017;7:43315. DOI: 10.1038/srep43315

[93] Zhu Y, Ghosh P, Charnay P, Burns DK, Parada LF. Neurofibromas in NF1: Schwann cell origin and role of tumor environment. Science. 2002;**296**: 920-922. DOI: 10.1126/science.1068452

[94] Mayes DA, Rizvi TA, Cancelas JA, Kolasinski NT, Ciraolo GM, Stemmer-Rachamimov AO, et al. Perinatal or adult Nf1 inactivation using tamoxifen-inducible PlpCre each cause neurofibroma formation. Cancer Research. 2011;**71**:4675-4685. DOI: 10.1158/0008-5472.CAN-10-4558

[95] Prada CE, Jousma E, Rizvi TA, Wu J, Dunn RS, Mayes DA, et al. Neurofibroma-associated macrophages play roles in tumor growth and response to pharmacological inhibition. Acta Neuropathologica. 2013;**125**:159-168. DOI: 10.1007/s00401-012-1056-7

[96] Yang FC, Chen S, Clegg T, Li X, Morgan T, Estwick SA, et al. Nf1+/− mast cells induce neurofibroma like phenotypes through secreted TGF-beta signaling. Human Molecular Genetics. 2006;**15**:2421-2437. DOI: 10.1093/hmg/ddl165

[97] Mirsky R, Woodhoo A, Parkinson DB, Arthur-Farraj P, Bhaskaran A, Jessen KR. Novel signals controlling embryonic Schwann cell development, myelination and dedifferentiation. Journal of the Peripheral Nervous System. 2008;**13**: 122-135. DOI: 10.1111/j.1529-8027.2008.00168.x

[98] Roger E, Martel S, Bertrand-Chapel A, Depollier A, Chuvin N, Pommier RM, et al. Schwann cells support oncogenic potential of pancreatic cancer cells through TGFbeta signaling. Cell Death & Disease. 2019;**10**:886. DOI: 10.1038/s41419-019-2116-x

[99] Armstrong AE, Rhodes SD, Smith A, Chen S, Bessler W, Ferguson MJ, et al. Early administration of imatinib mesylate reduces plexiform neurofibroma tumor burden with durable results after drug discontinuation in a mouse model of neurofibromatosis type 1. Pediatric Blood & Cancer. 2020;**67**:e28372. DOI: 10.1002/pbc.28372

Chapter 5

Surgical and Combined Tactic for Multi-Level Spinal Cord Tumor Compression in Patients with Neurofibromatosis

Vasiliy Korolishin and Yuri M. Poluektov

Abstract

Due to Evans et al. investigation, it is known that 26% of patients with NF II type involve spinal cord or nervous tissue tumors in the spinal column area. Although so many patients with NF have spinal tumors, not everyone has the potential to the neurological progressive symptoms due to spinal cord compression and not always tumors lead to invalidation of patients with neurofibromatosis. Unfortunately, a lot of surgeons consider that tumors required surgery and very often decide to remove a maximum number of tumors. Neurofibromas has different structural and growth patterns. Most of them has a fusiform type of growing. Sometimes surgeon needs to remove tumor with incoming nerve root with the risk of neurological deficit, or to perform intralesional debulking of soft tumor component, which occasionally leads to continued tumor growth. Furthermore, the decision and the sequence of the tumors removal rely on the leading cause of patient deficits. First of all symptomatic intracranial tumors should be removed, then intradural lesions. Certainly, patients with symptomatic spinal tumor need individual approach to the neurofibromatosis aspect. Decision-making needs to be accepted by neuroradiologist, neurologist, and neurosurgeon by looking at all sides of CNS imaging. So, it is important to make an algorithm for all doctors who try to treat patients with neurofibromatosis.

Keywords: neurofibroma, schwannoma, spinal cord tumor, neurofibromatosis, multiple spinal tumors

1. Introduction

Accordingly, our experience and literature date, there are a lot of patients with neurofibromatosis in the population, who need surgeon attention. Treatment of these patients' categories required very special access.

This chapter is devoted to important aspects of the diagnosis and treatment of patients with severe symptoms of neurofibromatosis. A small percentage of these patients suffer from manifestations of neurofibromatosis associated with the growth of tumors along the spinal cord. Often tumors compress the spinal cord or only threaten to compress the

IntechOpen

spinal cord. In both cases, it is necessary to differentiate the risks of treatment and the threat of a tumor, then offer the patient a solution that will be as effective as it is safe.

2. Neurofibromatosis type 1

2.1 Epidemiology, genetics, characteristics

The prevalence of neurofibromatosis type 1 (NF1) varies depending on population density and the level of the country's medical service development and is approximately 1 case per 3000 people [1].

NF1 is characterized by an autosomal dominant inheritance pattern. Key mutations in the NF1 gene affect the regulation of neurofibromin, which is structurally similar to negative regulators of the RAS proto-oncogene pathway. Thus, dysfunction of neurofibromin leads to hyperactivation of the RAS cascade, leading to uncontrolled cell growth mediated through [2].

The defining features of the disease include multiple neurofibromas and peripheral nerve tumors that affect the cranial and peripheral nerves, causing the compression of the spinal cord. In addition, chiasmatic gliomas are common in the pediatric population (up to 20% of all patients with confirmed neurofibromatosis) [3], gliomas of the brainstem, and spinal cord. Among adult patients with NF1, low-grade gliomas are widespread, and the overall risk of developing malignancies is 10–50 times higher than in the general population. The most common intramedullary tumor in NF1 is astrocytoma [4, 5].

NF 1, most frequently, manifests with dermatological symptoms, which include café-au-lait spots and cutaneous neurofibromas. Large studies focused on the frequency of the disease manifestation with various signs have not been conducted.

Thus, the true prevalence of the simultaneous occurrence of tumors of the CNS (central nervous system) and PNS (peripheral nervous system) was not carried out. Also, the incidence of multilevel CNS and PNS lesions in the general population of patients with NF1 has not been evaluated. However, our experience and the experience of a number of researchers suggest that multilevel lesions of the spinal cord occur most often, while one or several tumors can be symptomatic at the same time [6].

The overall cumulative risk of malignancy in patients with NF1 is up to 40% by the age of 50. That is, 2–5 times higher than in the general population. The risk of CNS malignant tumors developing is 40% higher, and the risk of developing MPNST is 1000 times higher [1].

2.2 Diagnostics

The manifestations of the disease can be very heterogeneous and depend on the age of the patient. The first symptoms that can be identified after birth are a cafe-au-lait spot on the skin, dysplasia of the long bones and orbital region, development of plexiform neurofibromas. Then, in early childhood, patients have an increased risk of developing chiasma and optic nerve gliomas, ADHD (Attention deficit hyperactivity disorder), and disorders associated with delayed psychoemotional development. In adolescence, the disease is often manifested by musculoskeletal deformities (including scoliosis), dermal and paraspinal neurofibromas, and brainstem gliomas. Monitoring of these patients should be systemic and aimed at early detection and regular control of the tumor growth of critical localization (threatening the life and health of patients). Regular checkups allow to detect MPNST and high-grade gliomas at an early stage [1].

Patients suspected of having NF needs regular monitoring, depending on the symptoms and growth rate of the lesions, these patients are suggested to undergo a full body MRI once a year/5 years, or a CNS MRI with contrast followed by monitoring for 2 years every 4 months and then 1 once a year up to 5 years (in case of CNS tumors).

2.3 Genetic testing

We recommend genetic testing to be performed at any age in individuals who meet the NF criteria. In addition, patients with an unusual NF1 phenotype, such as multilevel extramedullary tumors, should be tested (even in the absence of large NF1 criteria).

The global diagnostic algorithm implies observation by different specialists from birth (dermatologist, ophthalmologist, neurologist, psychiatrist), and the approach to neuroimaging and other examinations is determined by the manifestation of the disease in each case.

2.4 Imaging

It is believed that more than 50% of patients with NF1 have tumors of the internal organs, and therefore panMRI may be the method of choice after the symptoms manifestation. To detect intracranial or spinal lesions, it is recommended to perform MRI (1.5 T and higher) with i.v. contrasting. We recommend the MRI of entire neuroaxis regardless of the expected level of tumor location.

Full-body CT and full-spine X-ray in two projections can be recommended for progressive musculoskeletal deformity for orthopedic correction planning.

PET with FDG cannot be recommended as a screening method, however, when MPNST is suspected, it is the optimal method of investigation. In addition, PET can be used to determine the source of biopsy material in the case of progressive multiple tumor growth.

3. Neurofibromatosis type 2

3.1 Epidemiology, genetics, characteristics

For neurofibromatosis type 2 (NF2), the prevalence does not exceed 1 in 300,000 people. NF2 also has an autosomal dominant inheritance pattern and is caused by a mutation in the NF2 gene. This gene encodes a 595-amino acid protein called merlin or SCH, most similar to the exrin-readixin-moesin protein system, these are membrane-cytoskeleton scaffold proteins (i.e., linking actin filaments to the cell membrane or membrane glycoproteins) that act as critical regulators of contact-dependent proliferation inhibition and maintain the normal organization of the cytoskeleton by modulating cell motility, attachment, remodeling, and proliferation, thus regulating cell growth and development (tumor-suppressing function). Merlin regulates proliferation by acting through several cascades that include Ras GAP/Raf proteins (which regulate the MEK/ERK pathway) and PI3K/AKT proteins (which regulate the mTOR pathway) [7].

3.2 Diagnostics

NF2 is characterized by the development of vestibular schwannomas (VS); schwannoma of other cranial, spinal, and cutaneous nerves; intracranial and spinal meningiomas and/or other tumors of the central nervous system (eg ependymoma and astrocytoma). The most common intramedullary tumor is ependymoma.

Multilevel and multiple lesions are a hallmark of NF2 (MISME syndrome (Multiple Inherited Schwannomas, Meningiomas, and Ependymomas)). Multiple meningiomas are the second most important diagnostic criterion and occur in approximately 50% of cases [8].

3.3 Genetic testing

We recommend that genetic testing be performed at any age in individuals who meet the criteria for neurofibromatosis. In addition, patients with an unusual NF2 phenotype, such as multilevel extramedullary tumors and or extended intramedullary tumors, should be tested [9].

Otherwise, the diagnostic algorithm is indistinguishable from that for NF1. One of the main challenges for the management of such patients is the preservation of hearing in progressive bilateral vestibular schwannomas. The use of PET-CT as a diagnostic method fades into the background and can be used as part of preoperative planning for the removal or biopsy of CNS tumors. MPNST is uncharacteristic of NF2.

4. Treatment regimen for symptomatic spinal tumors in patients with neurofibromatosis

Extramedullary tumors often cause a decrease in the quality of life and cause disability for patients with neurofibromatosis. Dysfunction of the pelvic organs and impaired tissue trophism indirectly associated with tumors along the spinal cord can lead to life-threatening situations. Therefore, treatment must be timely. When meeting patients with NF, the clinician is faced with the problem of identifying the main and concomitant symptoms.

Treatment options include methods of local and systemic treatment of patients with NF. Local treatment includes surgery and radiation therapy. In recent years, drug therapy has shown significant efficacy against certain types of tumors.

The need for surgical treatment usually arises when growing tumors cause clinical symptoms. The most common is pain syndrome. If the tumor grows into the intervertebral foramen, along the nerve root, the pain is caused by stretching of the sensitive fascicle and has a burning and shooting pattern along the entire innervated dermatome, which increases with a change in body position. Local pain is usually associated with local tumor growth due to the involvement of the meninges of the spinal cord. At the stage when the tumor compresses the spinal cord, a syndrome of conduction disturbance is followed by paresis and dysfunction of the pelvic organs.

The priority clinical task is to determine the level of damage to the nervous system. So the removal of tumors nerve sheath tumor can significantly disrupt the function of nerve structures due to possible damage to the nerves adjacent to the tumor, which are the source of tumor growth.

In our opinion, an erroneous tactic is the removal of all detected neurofibromas and the attempt of the most radical resection of tumors leads to an aggravation of the neurological deficit and worsens the survival prognosis of patients with neurofibromatosis. Only tumors that threaten the patient's life or lead to an irreparable loss of function (paresis, dysfunction of the pelvic organs) are subject to removal.

Neurofibromatosis is a pathology that reduces the patient's quality of life throughout life, so surgical treatment, no matter how necessary it would seem, should not be risky for the patient's life or health. That is, the operation should not carry more risks than the disease itself.

This principle is dominant in choosing the optimal method of treating patients with neurofibromatosis and, in our opinion, is the only true one.

4.1 Extramedullary tumors

4.1.1 Neurofibroma

Neurofibromas are more common in patients with phacomatosis. According to our observations, neurofibroma is the most common cause of pain and more often leads to dysfunction of nerve structures in patients with NF.

Neurofibroma can be located symmetrically or asymmetrically in the area of the spinal canal or with an offset towards the intervertebral foramen and can be large. Often, neurofibroma has a confluent type of growth, namely, in the area of one localization there may be several nerves affected by neurofibroma, connected in the plexus area, each of which individually is a source of tumor growth and together they represent a large conglomerate of tumor tissue. **Figure 1** presents the patient with severe spinal cord compression by a dumbbell nervous tumor on the cervical level. In neurofibromatosis, both the first and second types, the phenomenon of widespread growth of neurofibromas is noted. However, this type of growth is more characteristic of the first type. Men are more likely to get sick, the tumor is more often located intradurally or intra- extradurally and grows like an hourglass. Relatively more common at the level of the cervical region.

Surgical treatment is the most optimal tactic since tumor resection is more effective in terms of local control compared to radiation therapy and intratumoral total resection with preservation of the tumor capsule. More often than in other departments, neurofibromas are detected at the level of the cervical spine and are associated with a higher number of relapses due to the frequent absence of clear boundaries and, therefore, the impossibility of total removal.

Surgical treatment should be safe for the patient, that is, focus on solving the main problem: reducing symptoms or preventing symptoms while maintaining the quality of life. Surgical approaches should be adequate to the size of the pathological formation. Our experience allows us to recommend a minimally invasive method for removing an intradural tumor or tumors at different levels. To create the surgeon's comfort

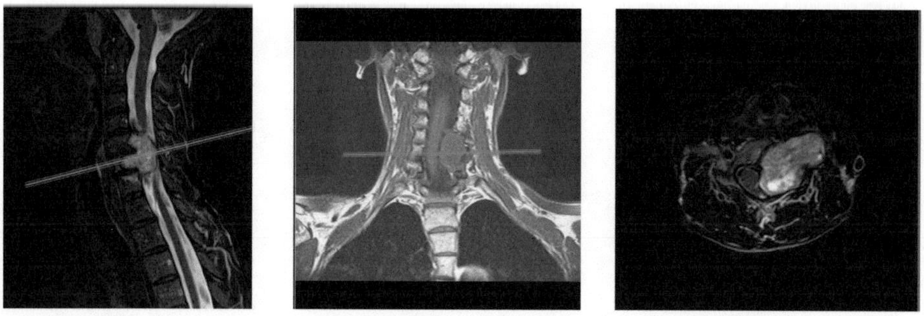

(a) (b) (c)

Figure 1.
Contrast-enhanced MRI of the cervical spine of a patient with an intra-extradural dumbbell tumor that compresses the spinal cord and extends extravertebral, adjacent to the vertebral and carotid arteries. (a) Sagittal view (T2W + contrast enhancement); (b) coronal view (T1W) and (c) axial view (T2W + contrast enhancement).

and reduce the risks of surgical trauma to adjacent nerve structures, the method is used to remove tumors of no more than 2 segments located laterally or centrally-laterally. If the tumor is located bilaterally or circularly relative to the spinal cord, it is desirable to use the posterior median approach with laminectomy. Laminectomy should be carried out taking into account the prevention of postoperative tissue edema. For minimally invasive surgical approaches, tube and telescopic retractors are used to view the bottom of the wound and dilate soft tissues. Analysis of the results of large series of operations suggests that operations are performed faster and with a lower risk of postoperative complications such as postoperative CSF leaking, intermuscular hematoma, soft tissue suture failure, superficial infection, or soft tissue infection. In addition, due to the absence of the need to skeletonize a large surface of the spine, the incision area hurts less, and the speed of the operation increases. So, the operation time is reduced from 40 minutes to 60 minutes according to various sources.

4.1.2 Schwannoma

Spinal schwannoma in neurofibromatosis is somewhat more common than in the general population, but the true prevalence remains unknown. In the general population, the overall incidence rate is 0.24 (95% CI 0.23–0.24) per 100,000 people. The highest prevalence of this pathology occurs at the age of 65–74 years, however, with neurofibromatosis, the life expectancy of patients is much lower, and therefore, it can be assumed that a large percentage of patients in the early age groups belong to patients with neurofibromatosis [10].

Schwannomas tend to grow intradurally and asymmetrically. Tumors grow slowly and rarely cause clinical symptoms until the size of the tumor is more than a quarter of the diameter of the spinal canal. Patients most often complain of local pain and pain in the extremity associated with a change in body position (**Figure 2**). If you do not conduct an examination and do not follow the path of local treatment, the patient feels weakness in the legs/arms within a year from the onset of symptoms, depending on the localization. Surgical treatment aims to reduce clinical symptoms and reduce the risk of tumor re-growth. In the event that the tumor is large, the method of choice will be intratumoral resection with the division of the tumor into separate fragments, followed by its removal without residue. Tumors that are localized in the region of the spinal canal from the craniovertebral junction to the sacrum become symptomatic when the spinal cord or nerve root is compressed.

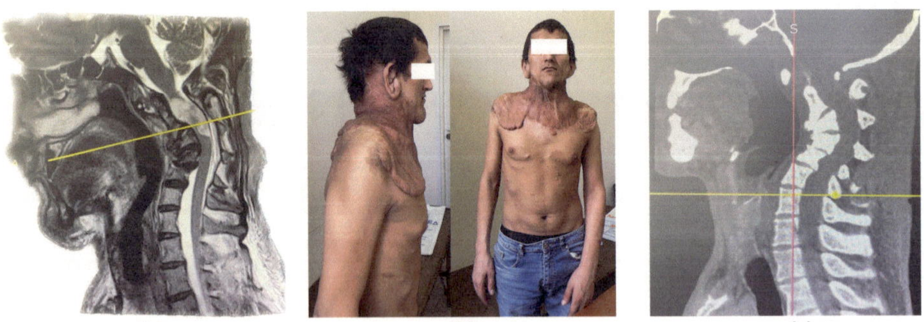

(a) (b) (c)

Figure 2.
MRI of the cervical spine with contrast enhancement in the sagittal projection: Dorsolateral intra-extradural tumor (schwannoma) with severe spinal compression (a). Patient appearance (b). CT 3D of patient cervical spine (c).

Type	Classification
Ia	Intraspinal, intradural tumor of <2 vertebral segments in length
Ib	Intraspinal, extradural tumor of <2 vertebral segments in length
II	Intraspinal tumor of >2 vertebral segments in length (giant tumor)
III	Intraspinal tumor with extension into nerve root foramen
IVa	Intraspinal tumor with extraspinal extension (dumbbell tumors) < 2.5 cm
IVb	Intraspinal tumor with extraspinal extension (dumbbell tumors) > 2.5 cm (giant tumor)
V	Tumor with erosion into the vertebral bodies, lateral and posterior extensions into myofascial planes (giant invasive tumor)

Table 1.
Classification of benign nerve sheath tumors [11].

Sridhar et al. proposed a universal classification scheme for spinal schwannomas. It can be used to unify the approach to tumor classification and optimize surgical approaches (**Table 1**) [11].

Total surgical removal with or without nerve root preservation is the gold standard of surgical treatment. Another treatment option for patients with small asymptomatic neoplasms is radiosurgery (CyberKnife) [12].

The risk of recurrence in surgical treatment is extremely small and does not exceed 6%. The main risk factor for local recurrence is Subtotal resection of the tumor, high risk of proliferative activity, and malignant histology of the tumor. Radiotherapy is a promising treatment for disease recurrence [13].

4.1.3 Meningiomas

Meningiomas occur in about half of patients with type II NF and often occur in multiple regions of the spine. In the study, it was found that cranial meningiomas correlate with mortality in patients with this disease (the risk of death is 2.5 times higher than in patients without intracranial meningiomas. Similar studies have not been conducted in patients with spinal meningiomas [14].

For type I NF, meningioma is not a common pathology, but multiple CNS lesions may occur [15].

The optimal method for diagnosing meningiomas is MRI with IV contrast. Without contrast, meningiomas are visible on T2WI. Calcifications are usually seen on MRI as areas of void. Occasionally tumors may be isointense on T1WI and T2WI.

An additional diagnostic method is CT. The tumor is visualized as a homogeneous, hyperintense mass with a wide attachment to the dura. On non-contrast series, it has a density of 60-70H. In addition, CT allows you to see calcifications, which allows you to make a more accurate diagnosis and simplifies intraoperative marking. For cranial meningiomas, CT angiography is an important study, as it provides comprehensive information about the tumor blood supply. In spinal surgery, this method is used extremely rarely.

5. Classification

The histological classifications of meningiomas can be found in more detail in the corresponding guidelines. When planning surgical treatment, the localization of meningioma relative to the spinal cord is of great importance, so they can be divided into several main localizations:

- Dorsal
- Ventral
- Lateral
- Ventrolateral
- Dorsolateral

In percentage terms, the incidence of meningiomas of various localizations very much depended on the specific sample, but most often tumors were found in the thoracic spine, less often in the cervical, and extremely rarely in the lumbar [16]. Menigiomas are often associated with other tumors. Currently, local treatment is the most optimal tactic.

6. Treatment

Most meningiomas are slow-growing benign tumors. With cranial asymptomatic formations of small size, you can choose expectant tactics, however, when it comes to multilevel lesions, it is necessary to immediately begin treatment. The effectiveness of irradiation for the treatment of benign neoplasms is still unproven, however, we suggest that in the presence of one or more small meningiomas that do not cause neurological symptoms (accidental findings), radiosurgical treatment can be performed.

Surgery remains the gold standard for the treatment of meningiomas. Removal of a meningioma should begin with the separation of the tumor matrix from the site of attachment, trying to preserve the tumor capsule, which is partially formed by the arachnoid membrane, as much as possible. The tumor matrix is usually vascularized. The tactics of removal depend on the localization of the tumor matrix. Dorsal and dorsolateral meningiomas. You should know that immediately under the dura mater is the tumor matrix. Therefore, the incision of the membranes must be carried out with extreme caution, starting with the outer layer of the dura mater. Removal of the neoplasm in a single block with such localization is not always possible. In some cases, to achieve radicality, it becomes necessary to excise part of the membranes along with the tumor. Especially in the case of germination of meningioma of the outer leaf of the dura mater.

6.1 Ventrolateral and lateral meningioma

The matrix, as a rule, is located in the root funnel zone. Often, the posterior roots of the spinal cord are, stretched on the surface of the spinal cord, and in most cases, it is possible to dislocate the tumor without damaging them. If the posterior root interferes with the removal of the tumor, it can be cut so as not to expose the spinal cord to unnecessary trauma. After the complete separation of the matrix from the inner layer of the DM, the tumor can be removed en bloc. This reduces the likelihood of tumor cells spreading along the CSF pathways.

6.2 Ventral meningioma

Removal of a tumor of this localization can be carried out by slicing, using not only microsurgical instruments but also an ultrasonic aspirator. Reducing the volume of the tumor avoids unnecessary traction of the spinal cord during removal.

6.3 Meningiomas with petrificates

The petrification site is resected along with the inner leaf of the dura mater. If the removal of the petrified part of the DM is associated with spinal cord traction, the affected DM is not removed in favor of subsequent radiation therapy.

6.3.1 Examination and follow up

With total tumor resection, it is possible to conduct dynamic monitoring with contrast MRI at intervals of 3, 6, and 12 months during the first year, then every 6 months for 2 years, then another 3 years with an interval of 12 months and every 5 years during life. If continued growth is detected, radiation therapy in the amount of 50–55 Gy is recommended [17].

For subtotal resection, the first MRI is recommended after 1–1.5 months followed by radiotherapy (the role of prophylactic radiotherapy remains controversial due to the continuing risk of recurrence) [16–19].

7. Intramedullary spinal cord tumors (IMSCT) associated with neurofibromatosis

Intramedullary tumors of the spinal cord are rare, mostly benign tumors, formed mainly from glial and ependymal cells, as well as cells of a different histological nature. Intramedullary tumors can lead to severe neurological deficits in the form of motor and sensory disorders, decrease, and loss of conduction function, which, in turn, leads to a significant decrease in the patient's quality of life or death.

With NF I and type II, the risk of developing intramedullary tumors increases. For NF I type, astrocytomas are the most characteristic, while for NF II - epindymomas. It should be noted that intramedullary neoplasms are an extremely rare disease, its prevalence, according to various sources, does not exceed 0.3 per 100,000 popula tion. According to M. Lee, Kuschel et al., the incidence of NF in patients with OMI is about 2.5%–3.9% [20, 21]. Data analysis of patients with NF D. Samartzis, M. Baser, D. Evans - IMSCT (ependymoma, pilocytic astrocytoma) occurs in 19 and 2.5% of cases, respectively.

The true prevalence in the population requires further screening studies. The survival of patients with intramedullary tumors varies depending on the degree of their malignancy, the five-year survival of such patients ranges from 28 to 90%. Gliomas account for up to 80% of all intramedullary tumors, among them the most common are astrocytomas (60–70%) and ependymomas. (30–40)%. Astrocytomas have a higher incidence in children than in adults, while ependymomas are more common in adults than in children. The sex-age characteristic of prevalence depends on the sample [22]. In 2011, R. Scott et al. published information on the treatment of 55 patients with ependymomas in NF-2. It is known that the risk of developing intramedullary tumors is higher in NF, but reliable statistics are not available at the moment. It is known that the risk of developing malignant neoplasms of the central nervous system directly correlates with the age of patients [1].

According to the available data, 20% of IMSCT cases lead to clinical manifestations and 13% have active growth without clinical symptoms. All this leads to the disability of patients. It is difficult to determine the degree of necessity and justification for intervention, especially in patients without clinical manifestations.

The gold standard for the treatment of intramedullary tumors is microsurgical removal using neuromonitoring [23]. The first stage of the operation is surgical access to the dura mater (DM), which is opened linearly. Then, access to the tumor is made through the posterior median sulcus (if the tumor is localized in the thickness of intact tissues; in some cases, a part of the tumor is located on the surface of the spinal cord and is visualized immediately upon opening the DM). The tumor is removed using microsurgical instruments under an operating microscope and neurophysiological monitoring. Tumor is removed within the morphologically unchanged brain tissue. The degree of surgical aggression is limited in the direction where the pronounced decrease in motor-evoked potentials occurs.

Treatment regimen is defined by the sum of clinical and imaging data. Recommendations for treatment are given by a neurosurgeon, a neurologist, and a radiation therapist.

In our opinion, the participation of a neurologist is necessary, due to the fact that patients with neurofibromatosis always have competing symptoms. Clinically intact intramedullary tumors need local treatment only if there is evidence of continued tumor growth.

8. Astracytoma

Astrocytomas are predominantly benign intramedullary tumors characterized by bad delimitation from the healthy tissue of the spinal cord. Astrocytoma occurs most frequently in adult patients and is the second most common intramedullary tumor (30–35% of all spinal cord tumors and up to 60% in childhood; 0.5% of all CNS tumors. Tumors are more often located in the region of the thoracic spinal cord (67%), followed by the cervical region (30%) and lumbar thickening and cone (3%).

In childhood whole spinal cord can undergo tumor transformation. In adults, a total lesion spreading is extremely rare. In rare cases when we see an adult with total spinal cord involvement we can assume the long-term persistence of the pathology. Cervico- medullary location is common for children and young people either.

According to the literature, 70–80% of tumors have the first and second degrees of malignancy (grade I, II), that is includes a group of low-grade tumors, 15–25% are high-grade (Grade III), about 5% are tumors of the fourth degree of malignancy (glioblastoma) (Grade IV). Thus, 20–30% of tumors are classified as high-grade gliomas [22].

Almost 20% of these lesions are associated with the formation of syringomyelitic cysts. The main surgical challenge is to find the tumor's "dissection plane" (the ability to separate the tumor from healthy tissue) for safe and radical removal. In patients with NF1, astrocytoma is most common in young men and rarely undergoes malignant transformation.

Generally, astrocytomas are found accentrically during routine imaging. Early symptoms are usually mild, leading to long and ineffective treatment. On MRI, a cystic component and poor contrast uptake are the most typical signs. Tumors can be visualized on T2W and T1-contrast series. The main imaging challenge is to differentiate tumor with demyelination and myelopathy. CT can be helpful to exclude ossified thoracic herniations resulting in myelopathy. The most significant sign is thevisualisation of the "mass effect" on MRI series (spinal cord diameter in the axial projection is increased in comparison to the neighboring area).

8.1 Nuances of surgery

There is no unified algorithm for the treatment of intramedullary astrocytoma. Surgical treatment of astrocytoma in patients with neurofibromatosis is complicated. Till that time when the symptoms appear, it is possible to discuss alternative therapy versus surgery. But the manifestation of symptoms often associates with big size of the tumor. And if the tumor was indicated in that stage, the surgery is not avoidance. The main problem of astrocytoma surgery is the absence of a transition zone in the region of the growing place – total tumor removal is impossible. So, facts and literature data indicate that surgical treatment is not absolute and does not predict good results. In the rule, as the main method of astrocytoma surgery is maximal cytoreduction or debulking. This method is the most effective for quickly increasing symptom redaction. An intact tumor in a patient with neurofibromatosis requires only observation, but if the tumor grows, radiation therapy is necessary.

Usually, the posterior approach applies. The millstone of approach is myelotomy through the posterior median sulcus. Good results depend on the quality and safety of myelotomy. Although identification of the midline is a difficult goal, it is possible by more wide laminectomy and the development of a healthy spinal cord area. It makes sure accurate midline identification and dissection with save of all vessels. In that case, if the tumor tissue is unidentified from spinal cord tissue, astrocytoma, as a rule, has poorly defined borders, and soft tumor tissue debulked by ultrasonic aspirator. This is the best method for reserving spaces inside the spinal cord creating. Some experts recommend debulking as treatment option if total tumor resection is associated with severe complications. It is desirable to leave a part of the tumor in order to avoid deterioration of the neurological status.

8.2 Examination and follow up

Contrast-enhanced MRI of the operation area is desirable to do within the first 24 hours, after 2 months, 6 months, 9 months, and 12 months, then, if there are no signs of progression, it is possible to continue monitoring at intervals of 6 months.

9. Ependymoma

Ependymoma is the most spread intramedullary tumor in population. Ependymomas account for 60–70% of all spinal neuroepithelial tumors. The average age of the patients was 39 years; these tumors are found more often (about 60%) in men. Basically, intramedullary ependymoma grows from the cells of the central spinal cord canal and looks symmetrically along its walls. In 25–30% of patients, ependymomas may have asymmetric growth of varying severity and spread laterally in the spinal cord. Tumors that are large in diameter can push apart the thinned posterior columns and come to the surface of the spinal cord directly under the arachnoid. Extramedullary growth of tumor formations is extremely rare. Ependymomas are most often located in the cervical region of the spinal cord. Ependymomas of the upper cervical spinal cord segments may extend into the craniovertebral junction and reach the caudal fourth ventricle. Such an arrangement is rare. Ependymomas do not rise above McRay line, and only syringomyelic cysts located above the upper pole extend the spinal cord.

9.1 Nuances of surgery

Ependymomas are more often available for radical removal. It is possible, by course tumor growing into the central spinal canal. Several evidence demonstrate that more aggressive tumors have less connection with the surrounding healthy spinal cord tissue. Therefore, they have great potential for gross total removal.

At the same time, tumors with a high potential for malignancy (Grade III) are more often complicated by metastases.

The posterior approach through the median sulcus of the spinal cord is most preferred. If the tumor is tightly adjacent to healthy tissue of the spinal cord, it is preferable to perform intratumorally decompression as a first step. Then the tumor poles removing.

9.2 Observation and follow-up

Contrast-enhanced MRI of the operation area is desirable to do within the first 24 hours, after 2 months, 6 months, 9 months, and 12 months, then, if there are no signs of progression, it is possible to continue monitoring at intervals of 6 months.

Too often malignant and aggressive ependymoma (Grade II-III) are complicated by local tumor recurrence and metastatic spread along the spinal cord membranes.

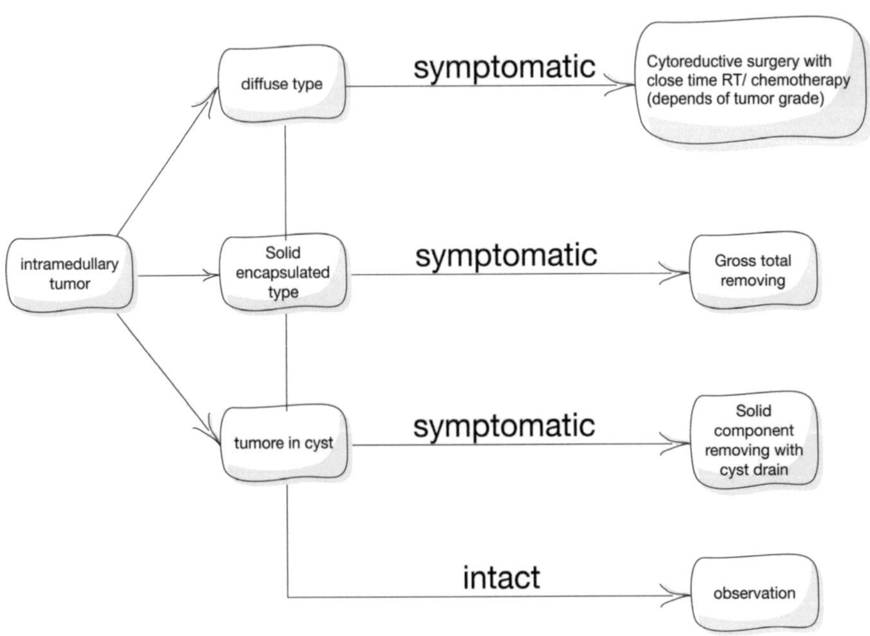

Figure 3.
Algorithm intramedullary tumors treatment in patients with neurofibromatosis.

So, if the local tumor recurrence/continued growth/spread tumor features or histological malignancy symptoms were detected – a radiologist's participation is necessary. Follow-up includes postoperative craniospinal radiotherapy, regardless of whether continued growth or tumor recurrence after.

Surgical tactics for intramedullary spinal cord tumor treatment consist follow algorithm (**Figure 3**).

10. Malignant peripheral nerves sheath tumors

MPNST is a rare complication of neurofibromatosis and accounts for 5–10% of all soft tissue sarcomas [24]. Frequency of occurrence - 1 per 1 million population per year [25]. Approximately 50% of MPNST cases are complicated by metastases within 2 years of diagnosis [26]. The majority of MPNST arise from peripheral nerves and nervous plexuses (sciatic nerve, brachial plexos truncs, sacral plexus). The incidence of MPNST of intracranial localization in the world population is less than 5%. The most important etiological factors in the development of MPNST are neurofibromatosis (NF) type 1 and radiological treatment for other cancers in history. MPNST is developed in 8–13% of patients with type I NF during their life [27]. In 10% of cases of MPNST appearance was associated with radiotherapy [28]. According to various observations, malignancy of neurofibroma occurs approximately 15 years after its detection.

The WHO classification of histological types of MPNST:

1. mesenchymal

2. glandular

3. epithelioid

4. neuroepithelial

5. triton

Clinical manifestations depend on the location of the tumor. The rapid development of symptoms is characterized (within several months), severe pain, and neurological deficits of varying severity. There are two forms according to localization:

- skin form

- deep formation

Too long time of observation and avoidance of surgery leads to metastases appeare may occur in regional lymph nodes and internal organs (lungs, liver, bones, etc.). Metastasis is carried out both hematogenously and lymphogenously.

10.1 Nuances of surgery

The main treatment for the primary tumor is en block resection. The main goal of surgery is to remove tumor. It provides the best result in terms of local recurrences and distant metastases. Localization of the tumor is very important, be the course of the totality of surgical removal depends on the growing place and relative of the tumor to surrounding tissue. The boundaries of the tumor are poorly defined, so often removal is partial [29].

The modern surgical approach to the treatment of patients with locally aggressive (without distant metastases) types of MPNST involves a complete cut of tumor. Thus, amputation of the limb, or very aggressive en block resection of the tumor within the margin of surrounding tissues of 2.5–4 cm, has always been considered the main method of treating MPNST. Alternative treatment as adjuvant methods of radiation and chemotherapy is possible but limited. So the view on surgical treatment has now not radically changed. For example, the location of MPNST in the limbs allows planning a wide gross total resection while maintaining the function of the limb. At the same time, this cannot prevent local recurrences or generalization of the process, since even the presence of an adequate resection margin is not a guarantee of total tumor removal. So early lymphatic metastasis is the indication for amputation of limb. The defeat of regional lymph nodes is rarely detected. Unfortunately, amputation is a limited method if the tumor is located in or around the spine.

10.1.1 Radiation therapy

Radiation therapy has become an integral part of the control of local recurrence in most soft tissue sarcomas (Suh JS) and can be used as adjuvant treatment or intraoperatively. But last publications show unhelpful of radiation methods for tumor cells of MPNST as to local control as in general spread [16].

10.1.2 Chemotherapy

Systemic medication treatment is used in the stage of generalization of the process, but there is no convincing evidence of effectiveness [30, 31].

10.1.3 Prognosis

The median survival time for patients with MPNST is 32 months [31]. The median life expectancy from the time of diagnosis, according to some authors, is 3 months. The causes of death in patients are usually metastases to the lungs and liver. Distant metastases (target organs - pleura, lungs, liver, adrenal glands, pia mater, cerebral hemispheres) are detected within 2 years from the date of diagnosis in 63% of patients. Overall 2-year and 5-year survival rates are 57% and 39% with treatment [31]. The frequency of local recurrences of MPNST is 65%.

11. Patients with multifocal symptomatic tumors

In patients with neurofibromatosis, meningiomas, and schwannomas appear with equal frequency. The sequence of surgical interventions strongly depends on the level of a symptomatic tumor on the spinal cord and brain tumors, in the presence of simultaneously symptomatic tumors at different levels, simultaneous surgery is not always preferable and a higher tumor is removed, or the one that causes the most threatening symptoms. Simultaneous operations are performed if the tumors are equally dangerous to the life or health of the patient. Presented lower algorithm allows to avoid risks (**Figure 4**).

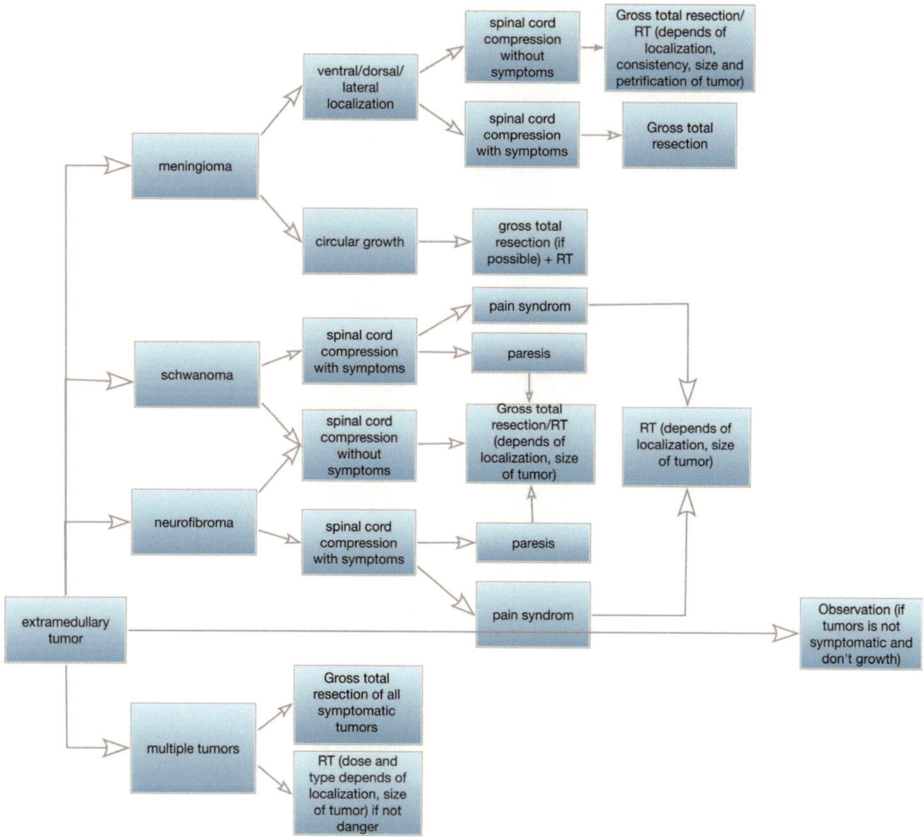

Figure 4.
Extramedullary surgical treatment algorithm.

Conflict of interest

The authors declare no conflict of interest.

Author details

Vasiliy Korolishin[1*] and Yuri M. Poluektov[2,3]

1 "AXIS" Private Spine Neurosurgery Hospital, Moscow, The Russian Federation

2 Burdenko Neurosurgical Institute, Moscow, Russia

3 Engelhardt Institute of Molecular Biology, Russian Academy of Sciences, Moscow, Russian Federation

*Address all correspondence to: vkorolishin@gmail.com

IntechOpen

© 2023 The Author(s). Licensee IntechOpen. This chapter is distributed under the terms of the Creative Commons Attribution License (http://creativecommons.org/licenses/by/3.0), which permits unrestricted use, distribution, and reproduction in any medium, provided the original work is properly cited.

References

[1] Gutmann DH et al. Neurofibromatosis type 1//Nature Reviews Disease Primers. – 2017. – T. 3. – №. 1. – C. 1-17

[2] Dasgupta B, Yi Y, Chen DY, Weber JD, Gutmann DH. Proteomic analysis reveals hyperactivation of the mammalian target of rapamycin pathway in neurofibromatosis 1-associated human and mouse brain tumors. Cancer Research. 2005;**65**:2755-2760

[3] Listernick R et al. Optic gliomas in children with neurofibromatosis type 1// The Journal of Pediatrics. - 1989. - T. 114. - No. 5. - S. 788-792

[4] Gutmann DH et al. Gliomas presenting after age 10 in individuals with neurofibromatosis type 1 (NF1) // Neurology. – 2002. – T. 59. – №. 5. – C. 759-761

[5] Strowd III RE et al. Histologically benign, clinically aggressive: Progressive non-optic pathway pilocytic astrocytomas in adults with NF1// American Journal of Medical Genetics Part A. – 2016. – T. 170. – №. 6. – C. 1455-1461

[6] Tonsgard JH. Clinical manifestations and management of neurofibromatosis type 1//Seminars in Pediatric Neurology. – WB Saunders, 2006. – T. 13. – №. 1. – C. 2-7

[7] Ruggieri M, Praticò AD, Evans DG. Diagnosis, management, and new therapeutic options in childhood neurofibromatosis type 2 and related forms//Seminars in Pediatric Neurology. – WB Saunders, 2015. – T. 22. – №. 4. – C. 240-258

[8] Martuza RL, Eldridge R. Neurofibromatosis 2: (bilateral acoustic Neurofibromatosis). The New England Journal of Medicine. 1988;**318**:684-688

[9] Campian J, Gutmann DH. CNS tumors in neurofibromatosis//Journal of Clinical Oncology. – 2017. – T. 35. – №. 21. – C. 2378

[10] Tish S et al. The epidemiology of spinal schwannoma in the United States between 2006 and 2014//Journal of Neurosurgery: Spine. – 2019. – T. 32. – №. 5. – C. 661-666

[11] Sridhar K, Ramamurthi R, Vasudevan MC, et al. Giant invasive spinal schwannomas: Definition and surgical management. Journal of Neurosurgery. 2001;**94**:210-215

[12] Konovalov AN, Golanov AV, Gorlachev GE, Kornienko VN, Trunin YY, Kotel'nikova TM, et al. Application of robotized system for radiosurgery CyberKnife for treatment of neurosurgical patients. Zhurnal Voprosy Neirokhirurgii Imeni N.N. Burdenko. 2012;**76**(1):3-12 (In Russ.)]

[13] Fehlings MG et al. Risk factors for recurrence of surgically treated conventional spinal schwannomas: Analysis of 169 patients from a multicenter international database// Spine. – 2016. – T. 41. – №. 5. – C. 390

[14] Baser ME, Friedman JM, Aeschliman D, Joe H, Wallace AJ, Ramsden RT, et al. Predictors of the risk of mortality in neurofibromatosis 2. American Journal of Human Genetics. 2002;**71**:715-723

[15] Goutagny S, Kalamarides M. Meningiomas and neurofibromatosis// Journal of Neuro-Oncology. – 2010. – T. 99. – C. 341-347

[16] Gottfried ON et al. Spinal meningiomas: Surgical management and outcome//Neurosurgical Focus. - 2003. - T. 14. - No. 6. - S. 1-7

[17] Golanov AV et al. Stereotactic radiotherapy for spinal meningiomas and neurinomas//Problems of Neurosurgery. – 2015;**78**(1):3-11

[18] Goldbrunner R et al. EANO guidelines for the diagnosis and treatment of meningiomas//The Lancet Oncology. – 2016. – T. 17. – №. 9. – C. e383-e391

[19] Yolcu YU et al. Trends in the utilization of radiotherapy for spinal meningiomas: Insights from the 2004-2015 National Cancer Database// Neurosurgical Focus. – 2019. – T. 46. – №. 6. – C. E6

[20] Kushel YV, Belova YD, Tekoev AR. Intramedullary spinal cord tumors and neurofibromatosis//Zhurnal Voprosy Neirokhirurgii Imeni NN Burdenko. – 2017;**81**(1):70-73. DOI: 10.17116/ neiro201780770-73

[21] Lee M, Rezai AR, Freed D, Epstein FJ. Intramedullary spinal cord tumors in neurofibromatosis. Neurosurgery. 1996;**38**(1):32-37

[22] Samartzis D et al. Intramedullary spinal cord tumors: Part I—Epidemiology, pathophysiology, and diagnosis //Global Spine Journal. – 2015. – T. 5. – №. 5. – C. 425-435

[23] Hadley MN et al. Guidelines for the use of electrophysiological monitoring for surgery of the human spinal column and spinal cord//Neurosurgery. – 2017. – T. 81. – №. 5. – C. 713-732

[24] Woodruff JM. Malignant tumors of peripheral nerve sheath buttock and lower extremity a study of 43 cases. Cancer. 1990;**66**:1253-1265. DOI: 10.1002/1097;2-p

[25] Angelov L, Guha A. Peripheral nerve Tumors. Neuro oncology foundation. In: Bernstein M, editor. Ms. Berger. New York: Theme Publishers; 2000. pp. 434-444 One

[26] Karmody CS. Malignant schwannoma of the trigeminal nerve. Otolaryngology - Head and Neck Surgery. 1979;**87**:594-598

[27] Brenner W, Gawad Ka FR, Hagel C, von Deimling A, de Wit M, Boucher R, et al. Prognostic value of PET FDG in patients with neurofibromatosis 1-type and malignant tumors of peripheral nerve sheath. European Journal of Nuclear Medicine and Molecular Imaging. 2006;**11**:1-5

[28] Amin SA, Flanagan A, Patterson D, Lehovsky J. Radiation therapy - induced malignant tumors of the peripheral nerves of the caudal tail. Spine. 2004;**29**(21):E506-E509

[29] Carli M, Ferrari A, Mattke A, Zanetti I, Casanova M, Bisogno G, et al. Pediatric malignant peripheral nerve sheath tumor: The Italian and German soft tissue sarcoma cooperative group. Journal of Clinical Oncology. 2005;**23**(33):8422-8430

[30] Action DV, PR R, Hornicek J, Gebhardt MC, Mankin HJ. Survival data for patients with malignant schwannoma. Wedge Orthopedic Relative Research. 2004;**426**:69-73

[31] Masaru F. Descended from Beppu g, Asanuma to Fuji K: A malignant tumor of the peripheral nerve sheath responds to chemotherapy. Journal of Bone and Joint Surgery (British). 2004;**86**(1):113-115